Motherhood by Choice:

Pioneers in Women's Health and Family Planning

Perdita Huston

The Feminist Press at The City University of New York
New York

Published 1992 by The Feminist Press at The City University of New York, 311 East 94th Street, New York, NY 10128

Distributed by The Talman Company, 150 Fifth Avenue, New York, NY 10011

Printed in Great Britain

96 95 94 93 92 5 4 3 2 1

Library of Congress Cataloging-in-Publication Data

    Huston, Perdita. 1936–
      Motherhood by choice: pioneers in women's health & family planning / Perdita Huston.
        p.   cm.
      Includes bibliographical references.
      ISBN 1-55861-068-5 : $35.00 – ISBN 1-55861-069-3 : $14.95
      1. Birth control – Biography. 2. Birth control–Cross-cultural studies.   I. Title
      H0764.A2H87 1992
      304.6'66 dc20   91-44239
                                                CIP

The Feminist Press is grateful to Genevieve Vaughan for her generous support of this publication.

For Marion Althea Brooks Huston to whose love and encouragement I owe all, and for Marcelle Simone Jeanne Melet Champey, who understood and practised sisterhood across cultures and generations.

Contents

ACKNOWLEDGEMENTS

I am particularly grateful to those who were willing to participate in this oral history. As the collector of these stories, I
feel very fortunate to have met and talked with those whose
words and deeds are the basis for this book. I regret, however,
that the wit and laughter of these remarkable activists cannot
be conveyed by the printed page.

Countless other individuals contributed to this book through
their counsel and suggestions and through assistance in
arranging interviews. Particular appreciation is expressed to
colleagues at the International Planned Parenthood Federation
headquarters in London: Rosanna Heralall was most gracious
in volunteering her time to translate Spanish texts and assisting
in research and contacts for the chapter on Dr Evangelina
Rodriguez. The research skills of Barbara Morse, and librarians
Rita Ward and Jennifer McHardy were invaluable in preparing
the final manuscript. Pauline Quinn provided invaluable administrative assistance. Dr Malika Ladjali, Karen Newman and
Frances Perrow patiently contributed their time and knowledge
in answering queries and discussing issues. Jeremy Hamand,
Rupert Walder and Paige Alexander were exceedingly helpful in
technical production matters. John Rowley's assistance with
publishing negotiations was invaluable.

Among the many people who welcomed me to their offices
and homes during the visits abroad I would like to express my
appreciation to the following individuals:

Asociación Dominicana Pro-Bienestar de la Familia, Inc: Magaly
Caram de Alvarez, Executive Director; Angela de León Navarro,
Director of Public Relations; Florissa Abreu, interpreter.

Swedish Association for Sex Education (Riksförbundet för
Sexuell Upplysning): Kerstin Strid, Executive Director; Norwegian Broadcasting Corporation: Mette Janson, Joar Larsen
and Haagen Ringnes.

The Family Planning Association of Sri Lanka: Daya Abeywick-
rema, Executive Director. Bradman Weerakoon, former Secretary General of IPPF; Malsire Dias and Nalin Fernando.

Singapore Family Planning Asssociation: Amy Tan, Executive Director; Pearl Lee, former intern in the Information Office, IPPF London, and a helpmate while in Singapore.

Alexandria Family Planning Association: Dr Salha Awad, President; Ines Shanan, Executive Director.

Planned Parenthood Assocation of Thailand: Sombhong Pattawichaiporn, Executive Director; Apinya Choonhahirum, programme officer.

Tunisia: Tijani Chaouch–Bouraoui, Director Arab World Region Field Office.

Family Planning Association of Bangladesh: Mukarram H Chowdhury, Director General; Manzrul Hoque Sarkar, Personnel Officer.

At the New Zealand Family Planning Association: Christine Taylor, President (also Treasurer of IPPF); Joan Mirkin, Executive Director, Ann Mehaffey and Rose Hart.

Planned Parenthood Association of Ghana: Nii Adote Addo, Senior Programme Officer, and his wife who shared New Year's Day 1991 with me; F.R. Nnoma–Addison, President; I.K. Boaten, Executive Director; and J. Samarasinghe, Mr Justice Amarteifio, Judge Annie Jiaggie; Mrs Peace Acolatse; and Dr Fred Sai, President of IPPF.

Japan Family Planning Association: Yasuo Kon, Executive Director. Japanese Organization for International Co-operation in Family Planning, Inc. (JOICFP): Chojiro Kunii, Chairman/Executive Director; Aiko Iijima, Programme Officer, who was my guide and interpreter; Mr Sayama who provided excellent photographs; and the gracious host officials at Nagano Prefecture and Susaka City.

Association Malienne pour la Protection et la Promotion de la Famille (AMPPF): Abdoul Karim Sangaré, President; Lansina Sidibé, Executive Director; Mamadou Moussa Doumbia, agent technique.

Lastly I would like to thank Dr Halfdan Mahler whose support was essential to this project and Doris Linder, historian and biographer of Elise Ottesen–Jensen whose knowledge and insights were invaluable. I should add that the opinions I have expressed in this book are entirely my own.

Foreword

by Dr Fred Sai, IPPF President

". . . the right to decide freely and responsibly on the number and spacing of their children and to have access to the information, education and means to enable them to exercise these rights"
UN Convention on the Elimination of All Forms of Discrimination Against Women (Article 16)

Over the years, thousands of individuals have dared question the status quo, defy customs, laws and what was socially "acceptable" to raise the issues of planned parenthood, contraceptive availability and sex education. Without the commitment of those activists, the reproductive freedoms so widely available today would not exist.

In commemorating the 40th anniversary of the International Planned Parenthood Federation (1952–1992) it seems fitting that we pay tribute to a few among those who promoted women's right to choose motherhood voluntarily, and who became the forerunners of the worldwide planned parenthood movement.

In so doing we wish to get a better grasp of the origins and the spread of the family planning movement, and of the pioneering work of women and men from diverse backgrounds, each with their own vision of a better future. For me, the interviews in this book hold a most important refutation of the allegation that family planning is a western imposed concept. I find this notion very patronizing. While, in many cases, future pioneers returned home from study in the colonial capitals with new ideas, those ideas met with a very real local need.

The IPPF member associations in 132 countries are voluntary groups administered by indigenous volunteers. They know and understand the needs of their societies. As volunteer organizations they can provide spontaneous and responsive action on a range of issues which government may not wish to address. They can fill the gaps.

Chapter 1
Looking Back to Learn

Shidzue Kato, the pioneer of family planning and women's rights in modern Japan, wrote of her friend, Margaret Sanger:

> She was utterly convinced of the righteousness of her cause: if poor mothers and their numerous poor children were to be saved from lives of misery, the message of birth control had to be spread.
>
> If women were not allowed knowledge to control their own bodies, they would never be free.[1]

The following chapters document the personal experiences of women and men who shared that belief and who dedicated themselves to changing society's attitudes to sex education and to women's right to motherhood by choice. Their efforts were always controversial; they met with hostility, public insults and physical threats, but they would not be deterred.

Their stories are presented here for two reasons: to honour those who dared challenge authority and convention in order to bring attention to the health needs of women and their families, and to prompt others to take up the struggle for reproductive rights. For, sadly, the right to choose when and if to bring a child into the world is a fundamental human right which is far from being universally honoured.

Two years ago, as the International Planned Parenthood Federation began to discuss possible publications for its 40th anniversary in 1992, reference was made to Beryl Suitters' remarkable history of the Federation's early days. *Be Brave and Angry*, written twenty years ago, chronicles the evolution of an institution's structure.[2] Now, it was proposed, it might be wise to capture the personal side of the activists' experience, the anecdotes and reflections which will be lost when the early pioneers of family planning are no longer with us. As a journalist who had worked for the Federation, I was asked to do this. The Secretary General of the Federation then asked each member association to nominate individuals to be profiled in an oral history, and a series of interviews took place from 1989 to 1991.

This is *not* a history of family planning associations, nor of the International Planned Parenthood Federation. It is a series of recollections of, or about, individuals who made significant contributions to the family planning movement. The intent is to discover, through these verbalized portraits, the motivation, strategies and heart-aches of past activists. Years after painful experiences, many of the interviewees recalled difficult times with a touch of anguish. Many sought to disguise their hurt with pauses, grimaces, jokes or playful comments.

Selecting those to be interviewed was not easy. Queries to family planning organizations resulted in over one hundred nominees. It was suggested that I limit the choice to those who had retired from active family planning work, and to notable activists who were now dead, relying on interviews with former friends and colleagues. In some cases, it was not an individual, but a group of individuals which enabled the introduction of family planning services. In others, a single forceful person was the key. Constraints of time and funds resulted in the selection of 12 individuals. Of the eight women and four men, nine were from less developed countries. Six of the 12 were no longer living. The interview format was chosen as a way of capturing recollections, feelings and views while it is still possible to do so. The ability to recall events was better in some individuals than in others, and some of the memories conflict. Several of those interviewed were shy and hesitant, while others spoke easily of themselves and of their work.

They are presented in order of their birth. Some began their work long before any variety of contraceptives was available and before the creation of the international family planning movement. Others benefited from the support of foundations, church groups, donor agencies and the experience of many committed individuals as well as the International Planned Parenthood Federation.

For each pioneer, the origins of their interest in family planning is different, their motives based on personal experience or tragedy. Each travelled his/her own path to brave public scorn, and to change attitudes and laws for the benefit of others. Each was convinced that women must gain control over their lives and that choice in matters of childbearing was central to this. Because of the diversity of backgrounds, cultures and approaches, the chapters vary in presentation and length. Those which focus on deceased pioneers, and which necessarily rely on the memories of friends and colleagues, are quite different in style from those in which an elderly activist personally recalls "the early days".

A book of this nature can barely scratch the surface of the history of reproductive rights. There will be readers who know or have met some of the individuals cited here and who may feel there is much more to be said about their work. That is no doubt true. Alas, oral histories are limited by what is actually said. I hope, nonetheless, that this modest effort will contribute to increasing interest in one of the most significant social movements of this century.

The contrast of personalities portrayed here is matched by the diversity of the situations in each country at the time of their work. In the developing countries, colonial rule was often still in force or newly independent nations were bound by laws inherited from the colonial power. New nations were in economic and social transition. Ethnic groups vied for power; social classes competed for the "benefits" of independence. The idea of limiting family/tribe/group size conjured up fears of weakening one's position in the new societies. Newly independent governments often took a pro-natalist stance believing that more citizens would make them more powerful.

In the industrialized nations, World War II postponed the social welfare agenda for over a decade. Official attitudes were greatly influenced by the war and its effect on family and population patterns. Fear of the Cold War's potential for renewed armed conflict favoured pro-natalist attitudes.

In the case of the Dominican Republic, a dictator's rule squashed all attempts to promote beneficial social policies. When the Swedish pioneer began her campaign to provide contraceptives, Sweden was a poverty stricken, largely illiterate, rural nation. Ignorance of the human body and its reproductive cycle was widespread. The enlightened prosperity Sweden enjoys today is in stark contrast to 60 years ago when Elise Ottesen-Jensen advocated sex education and contraception.

In just about every country, family planning and abortion had been available to wealthy women despite legal restriction or religious beliefs. With access to the best medical care, upper class women were able to enjoy motherhood by choice. They could obtain costly contraceptives and, protected by their social status, they were in no danger of prosecution for illegal abortions. The fact that poor women had no access to this choice was, in the eyes of many, an unacceptable injustice. Poor women were obliged to try all sorts of home made concoctions to avoid pregnancy, and when that failed, the more desperate turned to untrained abortionists, self-mutilation and suicide. The horror of deaths or chronic illness from septic abortions was the prime motivating force for the pioneers with whom I spoke.

In post-war Japan, Miyoshi Oba confronted an unusual situation. Abortion was legal but contraceptives were scarce. Ms Ohba's goal was to provide information and contraception, convinced that *prevention* of unwanted pregnancies was preferable to the *cure* of abortion.

The diversity of origins of those interviewed was remarkable. More than half were of the privileged class of their society, and had access to education and training and made good use of their access to the power structure. Others were of more humble origin and were rarely accepted by the medical or social establishments. The male pioneers were all medical doctors from developing nations and had studied in the universities of the colonial power. Few among their student-day patients had been malnourished, anaemic or married before puberty. Upon returning to their homeland, they found health needs vastly different from those in England or France. In particular, women's health was deplorable; if it was to be improved planned motherhood was essential.

These men were favoured by their gender; they studied, travelled and entered the seats of power far more readily than their female peers. As a result their experience is infinitely less traumatic than that of the women, who bore the brunt of society's unwillingness to recognize, or welcome, women's leadership.

Women pioneers in birth control emerged from a variety of disciplines: social worker, public health nurse, welfare activist, journalist and medical doctor. Because their work necessitated contact with the daily lives of women, they saw the physical, emotional and financial burdens women bore and learned of their longing to limit the size of their families – and of the risks they took to do so. Regardless of their social standing, they were insulted and threatened for speaking out, for mentioning human sexuality and advocating the right to voluntary motherhood. Far more vulnerable to public scorn than men, they were an easy target for those who opposed change or women's rights. Theirs was a constant struggle to maintain honour and courage.

Styles of leadership and strategy vary considerably. Soft-spoken Dr Barnor of Ghana worked quietly, building bridges with key personalities, carefully laying the groundwork for a family planning association. New Zealander Elsie Locke relied upon her skills as a political activist and campaigner. Experienced in public speaking and adept at defusing opposing views, Elsie was not always soft-spoken and never backed down when opposed.

Quiet coalition builders or forthright campaigners, each had a particular style which influenced their contemporaries. Each volunteered their time for the well-being of others. And each is revered by those who knew and worked with them.

In sum, the will to improve the poor state of women's health and prevent the tragedy of unsafe abortion were the primary motivations of the men and women who took up the challenge to provide family planning for their compatriots. There were those who realized that their nation would not be able to provide the benefits of development to its citizens if the population doubled every 20–25 years. A few foresaw the impact of population growth on the natural environment, on the finite resources available to support increasing numbers of people. Yet the main motivation expressed here remains the experience of witnessing the disastrous health consequences or deaths of women caused by unplanned pregnancies.

Family planning will always be controversial. It touches on the most intimate of human relationships and the power-sharing within those relationships. Women who can control their reproductive cycle are women who are less dependent, more self-assured, more active. The spectre of independent women brings fear to the hearts of those who would maintain their power and privilege.

All sorts of arguments were used to resist change. Family planning pioneers were accused of promoting promiscuity, of being unpatriotic, of questioning God's will, of distributing pornography and of encouraging pre-marital sex. Motherhood was endorsed as the supreme role of women, children acclaimed as "gifts from God", treasures of the family and nation. Contraceptives must surely be "harmful to women's health". Some expressed their fears more candidly: "What impertinence on the part of women to claim their rights when they are under men's perfect protection".[3]

The health and welfare of women, of mothers and children, were obviously not the concern of those opposed to family planning. Indeed, pro-natalist rhetoric did not take the next logical step and seek to provide poor women with child care, free ante- and post-natal care, free maternity care or maternity leave. Even the medical community sometimes joined the effort to **control birth control**. Doctors of the wealthy did not always see it in their interest that family planning services be widely offered at low prices or free of charge. Some midwives felt that their income would decrease if women could choose when and if to commence a new pregnancy. Several pioneers tell of this resistance, of the outright greed they witnessed. The medical community's position was crucial because, in most cases, family planning was considered a medical issue as opposed to an integral part of social policy, community development and maternal and child health (MCH). By "medicalizing" family planning, the power to control services fell to the predominantly male medical profession. There are those who point out that this in turn has disempowered women – both the clients of family planning services and the women pioneers who created them. The decision-making structure of family planning associations today often bears out this observation.

According to those interviewed, the principal source of opposition was religious groups, principally, the Roman Catholic Church. Decrying contraception as sinful, the Church has forbidden its members to work in family planning clinics or use contraceptives. It has failed to recognize that planned parenthood is beneficial to the health and well-being of both mother and child, that infant and child deaths in the Third World could be cut by at least 20 per cent (three million deaths annually) with effective family planning.[4] Its obstinacy has resulted in tragedy for hundreds of thousands, if not millions, of women and their families.

Today we understand that opposition to family planning and reproductive choice has evolved steadily from condemnation of individuals like those portrayed here, to sophisticated efforts to influence government policies. This is evident in even the most secular of societies. Because of this well-orchestrated opposition, the importance of political leadership cannot be underestimated. The past speaks eloquently: where national leaders dared speak out, results were forthcoming far more readily. Of all the national leaders of the last 40 or 50 years, Tunisia's President Habib Bourguiba stands out as one of the first advocates of planned parenthood and the right of women to control their fertility. He lectured his nation on planned and responsible parenthood and the rights of women as far back as 1956, far ahead of most leaders of our time.

Attitudinal barriers to family planning, of course, resulted in legal obstacles. Several pioneers began their work by organizing campaigns to change such laws. Without a legal foundation counselling, training and contraceptive services could not take place. Ignorance and lack of sex education was another formidable hurdle. This remains the case in many parts of today's world.

Some pioneers found that advocacy of contraceptives resulted in accusations of being the lackeys of multi-national corporations or of racist governments. Pharmaceutical companies, medical practitioners and donor agencies were suspected of using women as experimental "guinea pigs" for their drugs, IUDs or **population control** policies. Between 1971 and 1975, for example, approximately four million women throughout the world were fitted with the Dalkon Shield, an intra-uterine device subsequently found to be capable of causing severe infections. In the UK 100,000 were fitted; in the US 2.2 million women were fitted with the device, of whom 12,000 filed damage suits between 1974 and 1985. Seventeen women are known to have died. A court case found A.H. Robins, the manufacturers, guilty of negligence[5] and the tragedy is one of the most well-known examples of corporate irresponsibility.

When Helvet Tellawi of Egypt introduced the resolution proposing family planning as a basic human right to the International Conference on Human Rights (Tehran 1968), it was a revolutionary idea. Today that right is enshrined in half a dozen international covenants and conventions.[6] Yet powerful forces seek to deny that right to millions of women and men. On every continent there are attempts to curtail reproductive rights.

From Kenya, Zambia and Mexico come reports of increasingly vocal opposition to family planning from groups which appear to be funded by US or UK based anti-choice organizations. The unification of the two Germanies was delayed several weeks because of disagreements over abortion policy. The more liberal policy of the former German Democratic Republic was not acceptable to the government of the Federal Republic, the wealthier of the two, and a decision on abortion policy for united Germany was postponed until 1992. Singapore, which almost miraculously decreased its birth rate a decade ago, is now publicly criticizing its young women, saying they are "too well educated" or "too particular about whom they marry" because they marry much later than in the past.

The individual's right to manage fertility is a basic human one; the fact remains that an estimated 300 million couples in the world who would like to plan their families have no access to modern contraceptive services. According to the UN Population Fund (UNFPA), providing them with family planning services will necessitate an increase in investment from $4.5 billion in 1990 to $9 billion annually by the year 2000.[7] In a world where an estimated one million women die each year from reproductive problems[8] and in which one in every 23 African woman dies of pregnancy-related causes, surely this is modest investment. But it is an investment that is needed *now*.

While visiting Ghana to interview the people quoted in this book I met a woman who personifies the dilemma facing many family planning workers today. Peace Acolatse, a nurse and midwife, was trained at the Marie Stopes Clinic in London in the 1950s. She became an early volunteer of the Planned Parenthood Association of Ghana. Now retired and well into her seventies, she still practises midwifery. The town of Peaceville is a group of dusty houses scattered along a narrow dirt road. Its clinic is the second room of Mrs Acolatse's two-room home. Children, chickens and dogs gathered in the yard as our car drove up. Dressed in the white, starched uniform of her nursing profession, Mrs Acolatse greeted us graciously. We sat talking in her sitting room. On a bed in the far corner, a woman lay prostrate. "She needed somewhere to stay," explained our hostess.

> I can't be an active volunteer for Planned Parenthood anymore. Because of our economic situation there is no transportation, the funds are always lacking. I had to give up my car. It was too expensive, the petrol and all. It is a shame because now there is no transport to the hospital. Women come here for help often in bad condition. Sadly, I still see many post abortion cases. They need hospitalization so I send a child running, to ask someone to get a car. Sometimes they find no one to help.

Like Peace Acolatse, hundreds of individuals before her struggled in difficult conditions so that women might be able to enjoy safe and healthy motherhood. The stories which follow tell of 12 among them who worked selflessly at that task.

References

1. Shidzue Kato, *A Fight for Happiness*, JOICFP Document Series 11 (1984).
2. Suitters, Beryl, *Be Brave and Angry*, Chronicles of the International Planned Parenthood Federation (London: IPPF, 1973). Published to coincide with the 21st anniversary of the Federation.
3. Ibid.
4. Population Crisis Committee, *Family Planning and Child Survival* (Washington, DC, 1990).
5. Susan Perry and Jim Dawson, *Nightmare, Women and the Dalkon Shield* (New York: Macmillan Publishing Co, 1985).
6. See *The Human Right to Family Planning*, a compilation of international and national texts on the human right to family planning (London: IPPF, 1989).
7. UNFPA, The State of World Population 1991 (New York: UNFPA, 1991).
8. Jacobson, Jodi, L. *Meeting Women's Needs: The Reproductive Health Approach*, Worldwatch Paper 102 (June 1991).

Chapter 2
Andrea Evangelina Rodriguez
(1879–1947)

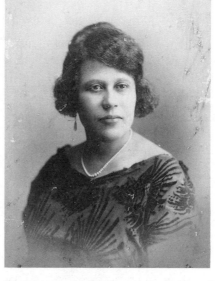

Dr Evangelina Rodriguez, the first woman doctor of the Dominican Republic, on her return from Paris, circa 1926.

Unappreciated in life and forgotten in death

Hispaniola, the Caribbean island shared by Haiti and the Dominican Republic, was discovered by Christopher Columbus during his first voyage to the New World five hundred years ago. Two years later his brother, Bartholome, became its Governor and founded the capital, Santo Domingo. Before the arrival of Europeans, the island was a land of peaceful native peoples who were easy prey for Conquistadors and zealous priests. Those who resisted conquest or conversion to Christianity were systematically massacred.

Strategically located on the sea routes between Europe and the New World, Hispaniola was coveted by competing nations for centuries. In 1697 the western third of the island was ceded to France. Over the next two-hundred years France and Spain struggled for control. In 1821 the Dominican Republic declared its independence from Spain. Overrun by Haitian troops within weeks, it finally gained autonomy in 1844. By the end of the 19th century the production of sugar cane, which relied on imported African slave labour, had become the *raison d'être* for control of the island by outside interests. As Spain's influence faded in the Dominican Republic, US business interests dominated its economy and political life as well.

At the time of the birth of Evangelina Rodriguez, the despot Ulysses Heureux was ruling the Republic. This rule by terror continued until 1930 when a general trained by the US Army, Raphael Leonides Trujillo Molina, became the dictator of the Republic following a popular revolt. His was also a brutal reign and ended with his assassination in 1961. Evangelina Rodriguez openly denounced Trujillo over the years and hoped to live to see him overthrown. Her wish was not granted, she died of hunger and exhaustion in 1947.

Evangelina began life with four strikes against her. Of African descent in a country which was barely emerging from slavery, she was also born poor, illegitimate and female, but by dint of her courage and will became the first woman to earn a medical degree in the Dominican Republic and gained further degrees in paediatrics and gynaecology. She also published poetry and a novel. She was an educator and feminist. Criticized and ridiculed as an eccentric, she was a lonely figure who fell prey to mental illness at the end of her life. Her work for the poor and her innovative medical initiatives set standards for government health care, yet she remains virtually unknown to contemporary Dominicans.

Dominican psychoanalyst, Dr Antonio Zaglul, had known her when he was a child. She had assisted his mother in the birth of several of his siblings. While in medical school, the young Dr Zaglul was assigned the task of writing an essay on the first Dominican woman doctor. "The more research I did, the more I became interested in this remarkable person, her intelligence, commitment and will to change society," he states. "I began to fall in love with an ever-generous woman; I followed her traces everywhere. My research became a labour of love."

Dr Zaglul and I met at the offices of Asociación Dominicana Pro-Bienestar de la Familia (PROFAMILIA). Now in his mid-seventies, Dr Zaglul arrived carrying a pile of documents he has collected which chronicle Evangelina's life and heart-break.

His biography of Evangelina is aptly titled *Unappreciated in Life and Forgotten in Death.*

Dr Antonio Zaglul

"Evangelina was born out of wedlock. Her mother chose to abandon the infant, leaving her to the illiterate father. He, in turn, passed her on to his mother. The grandmother made *gofio*, a sweet made from ground corn and sugar; she and Evangelina sold the sweets in the streets of their town. This was their only source of income in Evangelina's early years. The father remained indifferent to Evangelina. Occasionally he came to see his mother and the child but not regularly or in a way which gave her guidance. He was a manual labourer in the sugar cane industry, certainly not able to travel often or contribute much to the upbringing of a child. All her life Evangelina tried to find out about her mother, through the church or those who had known her. She had truly disappeared without a trace; Evangelina never even found her mother's birth date.

"When Evangelina was about 12, a neighbour Raphael Deligne, a well-known poet, was suffering from advanced stages of leprosy. He had lost his hands and could no longer wash or feed himself. His family was well-educated and respected but had fallen on hard times. His widowed mother could not afford to hire care for her son. The young Evangelina offered to help when she could. Each day she went to their home to bathe and feed Raphael. She did this out of compassion and neighbourliness for she received nothing in return but the friendship of the poet.

"Each evening, a group of Raphael's friends and admirers gathered at his home to recite each others' poetry and denounce government injustices. In the company of these intellectuals Evangelina learned about the world beyond her town. They, in turn, saw in her an intelligent, compassionate girl. They encouraged her to think of becoming a doctor. Evangelina cared for members of the Deligne family for many years. When Raphael died, it was Evangelina who bathed him. Fourteen years later, the brother Gaston developed leprosy; he shot himself rather than face the sufferings his brother had endured. Still later it was Evangelina who cared for the mother until her death.

"In Evangelina's childhood, San Pedro de Macoris was the most important city of the Dominican Republic. My father, a Lebanese merchant, settled there because it was a boom town; its port was the centre of sugar industry exports. Slavery still existed, even if not openly. Cubans, Puerto Ricans, Haitians and people from the British Islands were brought in to cut cane and work in the sugar industry. Blacks were considered the under class. White society was very closed. Even Dominican and American whites did not mix. Americans lived apart in the sugar industry compounds. Arabs remained together, as did the Spanish from Cuba or Spain. Everyone else was separated. The blacks, both educated and impoverished, were joined in a Negro society. There was a ladies' club for all black social classes and it is through the black women's organizations that Evangelina found early support.

"Primary school was free, and by selling *gofio*, Evangelina was able to pay for school supplies. But secondary school was a different case. The well-to-do people of San Pedro de Macoris had persuaded a young woman to come from the capital to create a secondary school for girls. It was an expensive school; attendance was out of the question for Evangelina. The new headmistress, Anacaona Moscoso, was from a well-known and respected family and she did not harbour the social prejudices of the provincial towns. She took an interest in Evangelina and managed to find her a job teaching adult literacy classes at night school. It was a remarkable opportunity. Through the intervention of the Moscoso family, Evangelina became a municipal employee, able to earn the costs of her education.

"When she completed secondary schooling, she continued teaching and in October 1903, Evangelina Rodriguez began her medical studies. You must understand that in those days not even the Spanish universities accepted women students. But through the intervention of those whose children she had taught or those who had known her through the Deligne family, Evangelina was allowed to study medicine in the Dominican Republic. Not until the end of the 1940s did other women begin to study medicine, perhaps 10 in all between 1910 and 1940. Needless to say, Evangelina's aspirations shocked many.

"When Evangelina had nearly completed her medical studies, Anna Moscoso died of childbirth complications. Before dying Anna recommended that Evangelina succeed her as Headmistress of the girls' school. Anna's husband was one of many who encouraged her to finish her medical studies despite her duties as Headmistress. This was one of the most difficult period of Evangelina's life: keeping up with studies, the school administration and then, once a doctor, establishing herself in a medical practice.

"Evangelina received her medical degree in 1909. She was

30 years old and the first woman doctor of her country. She soon realized, however, that it was almost impossible to earn a living in San Pedro de Macoris where the cream of Dominican doctors practised. She was young, inexperienced and a woman. She went to the town of Ramon Santana, opened an office and several pharmacies in and around the small town. She did some teaching on the side to earn extra money.

"The region around Ramon Santana was home to guerrilla resistants who were fighting the land-grab led by American interests. It was there that Evangelina first witnessed the cruel repression tactics of a colonel named Trujillo, who was military chief of the area. He simply killed people, whole families, in order to take their land. Evangelina denounced his brutality. From that time on, they were enemies. It was the beginning of an enmity which was to anger, threaten and frighten Evangelina until her death. The brutal Trujillo outlived the outspoken doctor.

"In Ramon Santana Evangelina's pharmacies were soon bankrupt; she gave free medicines to the poor even though the intent was to earn enough money to finance her specialized studies in France. Her dream was to become a gynaecologist and paediatrician. It wasn't until after the First World War that she was able to leave for France. The years of study there had a profound influence on Evangelina's political thinking as well as her medical views. She returned to the Dominican Republic with a specialist degree and many new ideas. The most controversial of those ideas were the treatment of venereal disease and contraceptive information for planned parenthood.

"Upon her return from France she discovered the frequency of the incidence of venereal disease. She began to visit the prostitutes' neighbourhood to offer them free medical treatment. People were shocked. They criticized her openly, 'How can she treat those nasty women?' Evangelina would not back down; she continued to treat prostitutes and would talk openly about it. It was almost boastful. 'Yes, I go there; they are not bad women, they are just poor women who cannot find other work'. The Catholic-dominated society condemned her. She became an outspoken critic of the Catholic Church's attitude to family planning and gave speeches about planned parenthood. When she promoted the use of condoms, she was publicly denounced by its priests.

"There is a saying in Spanish that 'All children are born with a loaf of bread under their arm'. Evangelina denounced such beliefs. 'That is a big lie. Children are NOT provided with food when they are born.' When a patient came to her with a second pregnancy she would say, 'Don't come to me with a third'. I won't see you if you come with a third.' I'm not sure she had contraceptives to give women – just the usual recommendation for *coitus interruptus* but, of course, that needed the co-operation of the man.

"Evangelina knew well the desperate situation of women's health. Her adoptive daughter is the child of a woman who died in childbirth. The woman's health was very poor. Evangelina had delivered her second child and had cautioned the woman against a third pregnancy; her life would be in danger. She gave her a supply of condoms. Two years later the woman returned, about to give birth to a third child. She wanted Evangelina to do the delivery. But Evangelina's prediction held true; the woman was doomed. Evangelina asked the dying woman if she could keep the new born girl for herself. Evangelina raised the child as her own; they went everywhere together until Evangelina began to lose her mind. The child was then about 12 years old.

"With the meagre earnings she accumulated, she bought old houses and converted them into homes for lepers or TB patients. At one point she owned about 10 treatment homes. She also started a free daily milk-feeding programme for children of the poorer neighbourhoods. Called the 'Drop of Milk', it, too, was an idea she acquired in France. But her tactics to organize the effort were certainly unique. One by one she visited the region's wealthy cattle ranchers. She asked them each for a daily donation of milk. She didn't beg or plead. She simply said that she needed milk for poor children.

"She was also involved in feminist activities in San Pedro de Macoris which was the most intellectually active town of the Dominican Republic at that time. The feminist group advocated women's suffrage and social reform; it published a journal, *Femina*, for which Evangelina wrote occasional articles. Evangelina's unorthodox ideas and projects led others to speak against her. But she was unusual in the sense that she didn't care what others thought or said about her. She had her convictions and lived by them. Her sense of humour gave her the ability to shrug off most mockery – most of the time.

"Two types of insults were levelled at her constantly. She was mocked as 'black', and 'an ugly woman'. She retaliated by emphasizing her blackness. The racist attitudes of the time tried to deny black culture; she responded by accentuating her African heritage. Rather than try to straighten her hair she braided it, piccaninny style. She dressed in materials which emphasized her culture and wore oxfords, men's shoes – not the high heels of the educated classes. Other insults were aimed at her womanhood. 'Because I don't have a husband, a man to protect me, they accuse me of being a lesbian. I get poison pen letters under my door. Even in the street when I pass by, people throw insults at me.' The accusations hurt Evangelina deeply. One day, she broke down crying to a friend, 'For them I'm either kept by a man or not interested in men.'

"Her patients didn't pay any attention to these rumours. They remained loyal to their doctor. It wasn't until several years later, when she became an outspoken opponent of Trujillo, that her patients began to avoid her. They feared reprisal if associated with someone who publicly denounced the dictatorship. In France her political awareness had been sharpened and she was influenced by those who fled the Spanish Civil War and settled in the Dominican Republic. She supported their ideas on agrarian reform and an agrarian bank system. She wrote newspaper articles and gave speeches calling for reform, knowing full well that the power structure was violently opposed to such ideas.

"Her opposition also took the form of poetry. She published nationalistic poetry in journals and the newspaper. Unfortunately most of it has been lost. She destroyed all her writings when she became mentally ill. She once wrote a novel entitled *Selisete*, the name of the adoptive daughter. I've never been able to find copies. Her books of medical advice, nutrition, hygiene and family planning – the books she wrote and gave free to her patients – they are all gone, destroyed.

"She gave away all her belongings, including the houses she had acquired as homes for her patients. The daughter was still so young she didn't even know about these assets. Evangelina's friends began to leave her, isolating her – because of fear, not because they didn't believe she was right. This was her greatest crisis – to be ostracized by people she trusted because of her political stand.

"Censorship was strict. She was watched, persecuted. It was not in her mind, it was real persecution, bloody and with a legal face. I believe it may have been at this point that she began to suffer from schizophrenic paranoia. I had trouble making the diagnosis in the beginning. I wanted to know if there was real persecution and what was the contribution of her illness to her perception of events. It is difficult to be sure because such a diagnosis is not compatible with her character. Her personality was not one to fall into victimization.

"Her life was very stressful but I don't think it would result in the kind of illness she had. At one point she was arrested and accused of being the instigator of a general strike, which could not have been possible because she was already subject to audio-hallucinations as well as other illnesses. When her illness became obvious to everyone, Selisete's father came to take the daughter. He was a Puerto Rican and, over the years, kept trying to get the child back but Selisete had never wanted to leave Evangelina. The child gone, Evangelina was totally alone; she began to neglect herself completely."

The following is extracted from Dr Zaglul's biography of Dr Rodriguez:

"She was weighed down with the burden of schizophrenia. She awaited her death with anxiety, this death which would release her from her pain. She was fed up with her delirious, vague, erratic thoughts which had brought her so much suffering. She would walk from Pedro Sanchez to San Pedro and Higuey, back and forth. When hunger overtook her, she would go to friends, eat half of what was given her and put the rest in a bag, not for herself, but for some poor soul. She had lost her reason but still felt for the underdog.

"In 1946, the sugar-cane workers challenged the tyranny of Trujillo for the first time in 16 years. They went on strike in all the plantations in the eastern part of the country. The dictator was surprised but recovered quickly and applied his usual tactics. He sent his most hardened men to San Pedro and La Romana. They chose several of the strike leaders and hung them. They were left hanging for days as examples to others but, more importantly, to limit the spread of strike action.

"The people were frightened. Rumours were spread about Evangelina being an enemy of the regime, a friend of the Spanish refugees; it was possible she was a communist and an instigator of the rebellion. They looked for her but she could not be found. An order was given that she be found dead or alive. Eventually she was found on one of her long treks from Pedro Sanchez and Miches. She was taken to San Pedro. Several days later, after interrogations and beating, she was released on a deserted track near Hato Mayor. This was the final nail in the coffin of the poor woman.

"Victor Canto, who saw her in the last months of her life, told me that she used to go to the Hato del Rey estate and crouch in a corner of the yard for hours on end without moving. She could not go on. She was taken to the home of friends. Two days later, on 11 January 1947, at one o'clock in the afternoon, she died in Rafael Deligne Street where she used to live as a child, just opposite the house of her deceased leper friend for whom the street had been named. I wanted to know the cause of her death and visited the Civil Record Office. I found that her face had changed colour and was told: 'She died of hunger and exhaustion'. What an incredible paradox. This woman, who for years had fought against children and peasants dying of hunger in her country, had succumbed to this very thing.

"She had dreamt of and achieved so much: dreams of a farmers' bank, her 'drop of milk' programme, pre-natal care for women, family planning, her fight against venereal disease, evening schools for workers and domestic servants, teaching child health, her maternity hospital and her small clinics for tuberculosis and leprosy patients. She was a woman out of tune with a society which considered itself to be cultured and liberal but did not understand the greatness of her spirit which she wanted to share with the community. She was rejected and for this reason, in the last years of her life, she chose to leave the real world which had been so cruel and inhabit the world of her dreams."

Francisco Comarazamy

Francisco Comarazamy is a journalist and editor who remembers Evangelina as a neighbour and confidant of his mother. His memories include seeing Dr Evangelina stop in the street to talk to a poor child or destitute man, then taking them home to feed and care for them until help could be found.

I went to meet him at his office at the *Listin Diario* newspaper. It is housed in a modern building in downtown Santo Domingo. A huge antique printing press dominates the lobby and interior courtyard. Mr Comarazamy's office was a jangle of piped music, radio broadcasts, air conditioning hums and telex machines.

"Evangelina strongly influenced the society and mentality of the Dominican Republic. Her commitment and goals were like those of Mother Teresa but she was not as religious as Mother Teresa and, tragically, people did not understand her. Her work had an enormous impact, albeit on a small scale. It paved the way for government social policies in the years that followed. Evangelina was a true pioneer.

"There were limitations to what she could accomplish. She had to depend on peoples' generosity which, of course, was never regular and dependable. She was obsessed with family planning and shocked by the comparison between Europe and our country. She was very conscious of the problems that a big family had on society and the country's development. Outspoken and non-conformist, she protested all the time against what was wrong, against the regime and social injustice.

"She condemned the rich and since we were living in a very strong dictatorship, a bloody one, she created a lot of fear that progressively isolated her. Since she opposed the government, the government made it difficult for her to work. She was very restricted in what she could accomplish. She wanted to open dispensaries; permission was denied. The government wanted to do that. Indeed, the government started delivering milk, opening medical dispensaries and hospitals. As the government took over her work, she was reduced to marginal activities and moved to small towns near San Pedro de Macoris which had no such services.

"She, my mother and other women talked a great deal about the plight of women in our society. Evangelina was not a real political activist. She wanted a better life for the poor and worked for social justice, but she didn't want to follow any particular political movement. My mother was originally from Guadeloupe and was a French teacher. She taught Evangelina to speak French before she went to study in Paris. When Evangelina returned, she moved into a house across the street from us. They became friends and remained close until my mother's death.

"She was quite good-looking, particularly when she came back from Paris. Well dressed, with feathered hats and all, she was actually attractive. She was always enthusiastic, for she loved life. When she began to do social work, working with prostitutes and providing family planning for the poor, she began to give up the fancy dresses. She became careless in her appearance. Her work with the needy convinced her that it was more important to be generous, than to be a fancily dressed woman. She began to neglect herself.

"At the end of her life she went from a dignified and self-contained person to being outspoken and critical. She lectured anyone she could about Trujillo; people began to think of her as a mad woman. She roamed around the countryside by herself, a lonely woman. She was incapacitated by her illness about three months prior to her death. By the time she died, she had lost most of her mental capacities."

Selisete Sanchez de Toribo

The day following the interviews in Santo Domingo we drove to San Pedro de Macoris to meet Evangelina's adopted daughter. Selisete Sanchez de Toribo is a small, serene woman, a grandmother with scarcely a line on her face. She was dressed in a simple cotton dress with a white lace collar, her hair cropped short. She recently retired after 38 years as personnel and purchasing agent in the town's largest pharmacy. Her home is a modest house on a narrow street, tidy and spotless. Selisete Sanchez was soft-spoken at first, but as the interview progressed she became more and more animated.

"Mother died when I was 12. I didn't realize she was ill; I thought it was just her way. When I was older I realized that some of the things she said or did were a sign of madness. But as a child I did not understand or notice anything strange.When we talked she always encouraged me and told me not to waste time on material things. To take care of what we had. She reminded me how hard her childhood was, about how difficult her life had been. She told these stories in a kind way, as a story not an admonition.

"Our house was in Calle Independencia; it served also as her doctor's office. It was a wooden house, there were many pictures on the walls, portraits and mother's diplomas. There was a huge cupboard with nice china and porcelain. All the seats were rocking-chairs, every one. There was a garden out back with lots of plants. Mother liked to garden. The largest room was used for consultations and there was another where the milk distribution was organized. Mother was afraid it would be given unpasteurized to the children if she didn't supervise its pasteurization right there, before distribution. The milk was donated by ranchers but mother paid neighbourhood women to help her prepare and distribute the milk. She gave them a wage. Many of them were migrant women.

"Mother was always proud when she delivered a baby, particularly if it was a difficult delivery or she had to travel far. Sometimes we had to go far out into the countryside, cross rivers, walk for a long time. I used to go with her and I know from experience it was a hard life. When the baby was born, mother would thank God for the new child and then teach the mother how to care for it. As a paediatrician she considered teaching child-care a part of her job. She taught sterilization, hygiene, how to clean the breasts before feeding the baby, all those things. She always insisted that mothers breast feed. Years later when she would see the child she would say, 'Look at the child, it is one of mine.' That is how I came to be her daughter. My mother died in childbirth. The labour was long and my mother weak. Evangelina told her, "Don't worry, I will take good care of your child". Since my father lived alone with two sons, Evangelina just kept me. Evangelina was a gift from God for taking my mother away.

"Whenever we visited the homes of families with many children Evangelina talked about the benefits of family planning. She said they shouldn't have more children than they could care for, or could feed. I would then see her give them a little package. Most of the time it was the women who wanted more information but the husbands, too, were interested to hear what she had to say.

"One day when I was about seven years old we went to visit a patient. She was a young woman but already had many children and had recently had a baby. Mother told her, 'You are still young and good-looking and can have many more children, but if you keep on having children you will become old and your husband will leave you with all these children. Your health will be affected, it is important to take care of the children you already have and yourself.' I then saw my mother give the woman a little package, but I couldn't see what it was. They were talking in low voices and it made me curious. One of the women's daughters and I wanted to find out what was in the package so we went and found it in the bathroom. They looked like balloons so we started playing with them. We were caught and mother scolded us, saying, 'Don't you know these things are important for this woman, for her life. They are not playthings.'

"Evangelina was a religious person; she attended Mass but she was not very friendly with the priests. She argued with them because they criticized her 'weird ideas' about 'things which should not be questioned'. She held that the devil could not exist. How could it be that someone more powerful than God could exist? She had many friends among the Protestant preachers. They gave her money and encouraged her work.

"When we went to visit patients she always talked about how bad Trujillo was, a dictator, a murderer and a killer. She told me that the day that he died I would hear all the church bells ringing. She said that she herself probably wouldn't see it, but 'you will, for sure, and then you will remember me'. Once she was arrested, during a strike; I was taken to my father's house and kept away from other children so I couldn't say anything about where my mother was or what she had been saying or doing. It was a very repressive time and people became afraid when she talked against Trujillo. The adults in the house tried to change my ideas about Trujillo; they told me he was a good man. I never knew that people criticized her. As a child this was kept from me.

"The first time she had hallucinations was at an official dinner in Santo Domingo. She was taken home by somebody. She was out of her mind, crying and screaming 'They're coming to catch me'. Her friends confirmed that she drank only one glass of wine, but mother thought something, a drug, was put in the glass. She didn't remember a lot. From the time mother was seriously ill until her death, I lived with my father. Evangelina brought me to him, saying that she was going on a trip which was not safe for me to go on. That was about one and a half years before she died.

"During her life Evangelina received no recognition for her hard work. Because she was so effective, she was feared by the dictatorship and didn't receive any official co-operation. They disliked her because she was an educator, a social activist as well as a doctor.

"The most important thing I learned from my mother was to love all children. She used to say, 'Mothers should give love to all children, not just the children born to them, but all the children of the world'. I, myself, raised three children who were not my own. I gave birth to three boys and then, remembering what mother had said, I decided to adopt three girls. I gave them an education; they all went to university. I taught them what I learned from my mother – to give the gift of love to all children. Two are medical doctors, one is a teacher. They chose those professions by themselves – perhaps as a tribute to their grandmother."

Andrea Evangelina Rodriguez

1879   Born in Higuey, Dominican Republic
1902   Graduated from Girls' Secondary School, San Pedro de
         Macoris
1907   Headmistress of Girls Secondary School
1909   Received Medical degree, University of the Domincan
         Republic
1915   Published novel, *Grains of Pollen* (lost)
1921–25 Studied at the Faculty of Medicine, University of Paris
         received advanced degrees in gynaecology, obstetrics
         and paediatrics
1947   Died (age 68) of hunger, exhaustion and mental illness,
         San Pedro de Macoris

Chapter 3
Elise Ottesen-Jensen
1886–1973

*I dream of the day when every child that is born is welcome,
when men and women are equal and sexuality is an expression
of intimacy, pleasure and tenderness.*
Elise Ottesen-Jensen, 1933

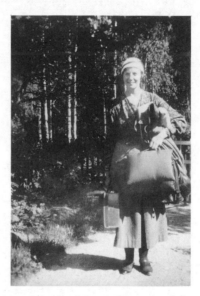

*Elise Ottesen-Jensen travelled throughout rural Sweden to counsel
women on family planning. Circa 1930.*

It is hardly conceivable that little more than half a century
ago Sweden and Norway, countries which today are models of
the modern welfare state, were afflicted with endemic poverty,
malnutrition and high maternal mortality. In the 19th century
their populations had increased rapidly due to "peace, the
vaccine against smallpox and the cultivation of potatoes".
Dependent upon the export of a few products (timber, corn,
fish) and subsistence farming, the nation witnessed rapid
expansion of a vast landless population dependent on farm

labour or domestic employment. Widespread poverty ensued.

Between 1815 and 1939, 1.25 million Swedes and 0.85 million Norwegians emigrated to America.

It was in this period that Elise Ottesen-Jensen was born, the seventeenth of 18 children of a clergyman and his wife living on the west coast of Norway. Through her mother's experiences and those of women in the poor fishing communities, Elise witnessed early in her childhood the difficulties of women's lives, fraught with poverty, ill health, constant childbearing and fatigue.

Women lived in terror of unwanted pregnancies. In the 1920s and 30s, ten to twenty thousand illegal abortions were performed each year. And yet the law was clear: the Contraception Law of 1910 decreed punishment for "Whosoever publicly exhibits or displays objects intended for indecent purposes or to prevent the consequences of sexual intercourse."

Ottar, the name the young journalist Elise Ottesen adopted as a pen name when she covered the 1912 Stockholm Olympic Games, considered these laws unjust and sexist, legislated by well-to-do parliamentarians, to the disadvantage of working women. A writer, lecturer and campaigner for women's rights, Ottar was particularly concerned about unplanned pregnancies and about sex education. An unmarried younger sister had been banished in disgrace to hide her pregancy and give birth far from home. To Ottar, it seemed clear that the innocents were being punished.

She founded the Swedish Association for Sex Education (RFSU) in 1933, and was one of the founders of the International Planned Parenthood Federation. A charismatic speaker, she travelled throughout the world, promoting planned parenthood and, above all, early sex-education. Without a doubt, she is the best known of the family planning pioneers profiled in this book. Throughout the IPPF she is recognized as one of its most devoted and dynamic members. As its second president, she was instrumental in building the movement in the less developed countries.

When I was in Oslo in 1990, the Norwegian Broadcasting Corporation kindly invited me to watch a filmed interview which was conducted by the well-known journalist Haagen Ringnes in 1966. Ottar was then 80 years old. Because it is a view of her life in her own words, I asked if it could be reprinted here. Authorization was accorded by Norsk Rikskringkasting and we are most grateful to them and to Mr Ringnes for permitting the use of this document. We have incorporated his questions with

Mrs Ottesen-Jensen's answers so as to conform to the format used throughout this oral history.

Elise Ottesen-Jensen

"I grew up in the incredibly beautiful coastal region of Jaaren. There were only long, long moors, covered with heather, that were quite purple in the autumn evenings. Colour that is stamped on my memory, and which, in itself, created happiness. It isn't easy to characterize the lifestyle of the region in words. But I would say that, in my earliest childhood, it was such that one was very careful about what one said and what one did, because everything was regarded as sin.

"But my family was not as pietistic as most. I don't think there were many clergymen's homes in those days that were as unbiased or as filled with happiness as our home was, or in which the parents had so great an understanding of the necessity of children being allowed to enjoy themselves. We were allowed to dance, we were even allowed to attend dancing school. We were allowed to take part in the meagre pleasures that were offered in Sandnes at that time. In our home there was a lot of music and singing, and father and mother were with the children a lot. There was a solidarity between the generations from which we could learn something today.

Both my parents were strong personalities – each in their own way. Father had an exuberant personality. Everything he got hold of became legends. Mother was the 'still water that runs deep'. Father was a great orator, but it was mother who quietly put everything in its proper perspective.

"It was that childhood which determined the course of my interests later in life, certainly. Among other things, I was very close to a young girl who became an unwed mother, and was sent away from home to another country. All her grief remained fixed in my mind, so to speak. I had a feeling of guilt, because nothing was done in matters like these. The fact that one could, somehow, keep young girls ignorant of sexual life and everything surrounding it – the fact that they knew nothing about what it was like to give birth or anything. I dare say this had a great deal to do with the direction my life took. Above all, perhaps, it is the reason that I took the initiative in creating a home, a real home for unwed mothers in Sweden. We have had 1,600 children there.

"Originally I had wanted to be a dentist. But there was an explosion, and I lost so many fingers that I couldn't be one.

I became a stenographer at the Storting (Parliament), but it was much too boring to imagine doing for long so I went in for journalism. It was very rewarding, and I started on the *Nidaros* newspaper in Trondheim. As a journalist, I sat in on the election discussions. In those days, in Norway, there were heated discussions about the new laws regulating the right to use natural resources. The Left did not want Norway to sell her natural resources to foreigners. But, during the discussions, I heard that the Social Democrats didn't want them to be sold to Norwegian capitalists, either. They should be the property of the people. These ideas moved me, so I became politically active in the Norwegian Labour movement. Martin Tranmael had just come home from America with new radical ideas. Everything that was radical interested me. I wanted change, for things not to stand still.

"When I went to work in Bergen I started giving lectures on peace and began organizing women. Oh, they were so badly paid in those days and things were so difficult for them in every possible way. I wanted to organize them, to see to it that they were better off. Those working-class women who came and listened to me, they didn't ask questions about what they could do about peace, or how to organize themselves. They came to me to ask about sexual matters. They would say something like: 'She, who knows so much, can she tell us why it is that the rich wives don't have as many children as we do? She, who knows so much'. I didn't know anything myself. Nothing. I just had to say, 'I'll try to find out for you.'

"And I did find out. First a little bit here at home, and later abroad. I came back with it. But, in the meantime, I had met my husband. He was also a fighter for peace, a syndicalist; he was an editor in Stockholm. So I moved to Stockholm and started working with family planning there. I travelled in rural areas, into the forests. Oh, how I travelled! If one could count the number of beds I have slept in! Or the number of fleas and lice and bedbugs I've been bitten by! But I lived the way the farmers lived; it was the only way to be accepted as one of them. When I came to a place where I was going to talk, they would say: 'Who would put such a fine lady from Stockholm up for the night?' But when I spoke, I spoke about their lives. Everything I said I had learned from them when living with them. I talked about how difficult it was for mothers at home. For the men as well. As soon as that happened, there was no question about where I was to sleep that night. They came and invited me to this place and that place. The next day their kitchen became the place to meet all the women who wanted to ask questions.

"I saw so much poverty, so many social tragedies. Incredible. I have been in cabins that were built right down to the ground, without a cornerstone, where the walls froze at night. In the daytime they thawed out in the sun, and this was absorbed by the walls. There the children were lying on rags in rough crates. And it often happened that when the husband crawled out of the bed, I crawled in beside the wife. When the lamp was extinguished, and the children asleep, then came the grief. It was then I heard I could help the woman.

"This was Sweden – the developing country Sweden. The Sweden of the poor. In many cases, when the bigger children went to school in the morning, the little ones had to stay in bed, because they didn't have any clothes – the bigger children had to wear them. When they came home from school, the bigger children had to do their arithmetic in bed so the little ones could put on the clothes and go outside.

"At the time Swedish law was anything but liberal when it came to legislation about contraception and abortions. As far as contraceptives were concerned, it was not permitted to show or recommend such methods. It was forbidden to have anything to do with them at all. Strangely enough, it was permitted to sell them. But nothing else was permitted. The law was the same here in Norway. When I travelled about, policemen often sat in the first row. It wasn't easy, as you can imagine. Those who had arranged the meetings, the workers, would come up and say, 'You have to be careful here. The police are very . . .' Well, what could I do then? I went on, and I talked about the difficulties of the people, difficulties with which these policemen had grown up. I talked about how difficult it had been for their mothers. They recognized all of it and were moved. When they were moved, they didn't take any more notes. Then I could talk about the other things. That's the way I did it.

"Before I started speaking, I would say something like, 'Now you must pay close attention to everything, because it could happen that what I say will be repeated in a different way than I say it. If anything is said that I haven't said, or repeated in a different way from the way I have said it, then I will need witnesses. Do you understand? So now you must all listen care-fully.' From then on it wasn't easy for the police to take notes. Now all that has changed. That's what is so fantastic. When you travel up through these forests now, you see lovely houses, painted and pretty, and connected up to water, and everything.

It makes one so happy to see the change for the better.

"Once I experienced something quite fantastic. It was around the end of the 1950s. A policeman had invited me to come up and speak in his district. Following the talk, late at night, I was to be driven to where I could catch the train at five o'clock in the morning. We were sitting in the car, in the snow; it was very cold. I said to him 'It was very kind of you to drive me down at night, when you've had so many other things to do today.' He replied, 'It's a pleasure. After all this is your car.' 'My car? What do you mean?' 'Yes,' he said. 'Do you remember what it was like for mother and father? We were so many children, and we couldn't have anything at all? And how worn out mother was in the past? But then you came up here, and you taught us youngsters what to do. And we only have two children. We've been able to give them an education. Have you seen how young my wife is? That's something quite different from mother. And that's what's so wonderful.' That time it was I who was touched.

"I founded the National League for Sex Guidance in 1933, and then helped publish a periodical for sex guidance. I conducted an extensive campaign for guidance in this area. You see, there was a great deal of prejudice to overcome. It was due to the fact that, previously, in questions about sex no one discussed it, too many people lived in ignorance. Even today, unfortunately, many are to be pitied. The question of sex, the fact that two people who love each other, also live together sexually – this seemed to be encumbered with shame. Parents couldn't talk with their children. There are still many who can't. When the child asked, they couldn't tell them how they had been born. They just said, 'Be quiet' or 'You'll find out about that when you're grown'. They tell the child that 'Morsan brought you in a box', or something like that. In Swedish the midwife is sometimes called 'Morsan'.

"We started sex instruction in the schools. It became obligatory in 1945. We instruct children who are seven, then those 11, 14, and 16. According to how much they are able to understand, we select what is suitable for them. But there are still parents who are afraid of this. They don't know what it's all about. They think it's something different from what it is because they, themselves, are so filled with feelings of shame.

"When I come to a place where I'm going to meet with teachers, I try to meet with the parents on the previous evening. I say, 'Tomorrow I'm going to tell your children this and that,

and thus and so. What have you told them?' I try to establish
contact between the home and the school. Then I can have five
hundred teachers who sit and listen, while I instruct children
of various ages. Then I talk with them afterwards because, if the
school says one thing and the parents say another – that it was
brought by the midwife, for example – and the school tells how it
really happens, then the child is the one who is left in the lurch
between these two views. Whom are they to believe? One can
shake their faith in their parents, and one can shake their faith
in the school.

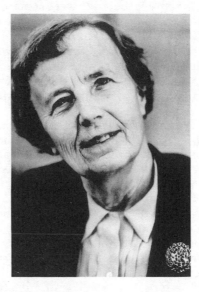

*Elise Ottesen-Jensen as President of the Swedish Association for
Sex Education (RFSU). Circa 1930.*

"The parents usually co-operate, even the ones who are afraid
in advance. That's what's so very interesting to see. When I
teach, I instruct them as if they were seven years old. Then I
can ask afterwards, is there anything you think that I shouldn't
have said? There were occasions when the parents had decided
in advance that they didn't want the instruction. I succeeded
in coming and presenting the lecture. It turns out that they
thought it would be something different from what it was.
When they heard me they understood it was all right for their
children.

"I say, 'Once you were a tiny speck. Oh, you were so tiny. You were like a speck of dust. You were lying in a teeny weeny egg, inside your Mother. And Papa – he has some tiny cells, as we call them, that can bring that tiny speck to life, so that a child begins to wake up. And Papa and Mama are made so that they can carry that little cell, the sperm cell, from one to the other. It can wriggle along. Papa can carry it to the opening down there, that all Mothers have, so the tiny cell is able to come in, and so that a little baby is able to come out when it's ready.

" 'And when the tiny cell from your Papa went in, and met the teeny weeny speck in the little egg inside your Mother, then you started to grow there. And you grew and grew. And then two eyes started to grow, and a little nose, and then arms and legs grew out, and hands and feet and fingers and toes with nails on them. And then came hair, and then you were a little baby. And do you know – one night Mama felt you move in there. Then she had to tell Papa: "I'm certain that we're going to have a baby, because I can feel it kicking and it wants to come out," she says. That night they lie awake for a long time, wondering whether it's going to be a little girl or a little boy. They didn't find this out for a long time, because you had to grow much bigger. 'And you grew and you grew. And when you grew, the little bag in which you were lying snug and warm inside Mother, also grew. And soon Mother's stomach began to grow, and became so big that everyone could see that she was going to have a baby. And I dare say that you can imagine that it wasn't so easy to be Mother then. When she wanted to sleep, you started to kick. Yes, and she had to carry you both night and day.

" 'But one day she could feel that you were now so big that you wanted to come out. And so she said to Papa, Now we have to find someone to help us get this tiny baby out. And so they went to the maternity hospital, and there the doctor helped you come out through the opening that all Mothers have down there. And when you came out, Mother put you to her breast, and there you got milk. And then you kept on growing and growing, and today you're so big that you can go for a walk in the woods.'

"The children love these stories; they're so delightful. It's not the children who are at fault, *we're* the ones who are fault. We must help them so they don't regard these things in the wrong light when they grow up. That said, I still believe that sex instruction should begin in the home, *not* in school. It should begin when a child asks: 'Where did I come from?' Then Father and Mother should tell the truth as it is – a thousand times more beautiful than all the fairy tales or all the tiny lies they can think up.

When I look back at my life there are very great changes in the moral climate. When I first went to rural areas, for example, the curtains were drawn aside in order that they could have a look at this immoral person who was wandering about out there. What did she really look like? Today I am given honorary degrees at the University, an honorary doctorate. I received the King's medal – not that I've worn it – the fact is that such change has taken place.

"I remember that *Dagens Nyheter* (The Swedish Daily News) asked me on one of these occasions, 'What are you particularly happy about?' I replied that I was happy that the sex question has become *comme il faut*. Until things are given their proper names, and until we can speak openly about such matters, the way you and I do, then they will continue to be encumbered with shame. We must bring them out into the open. That is the point. As fundamental as these questions are, they are questions about life. human life about human happiness. Believe me.

"Now it is the turn of the developing countries. It is very strange. When I am in the developing countries – I have worked in Asia and Africa and other parts of the world – I see how the people get along there. In reality it's Norway and Sweden all over again. The same as it was when I started years ago. The same funny youngsters. The same filth. The same shortages of food and clothing. There's the same lack of the slightest cultural advantages. It's just that everything is on a much grander scale. I had thought that it would be difficult to talk about such questions in the developing countries. Naturally, there are difficulties, but we don't have the religious difficulties that we had anticipated. The religious difficulties that we have to deal with are largely Catholicism. When the Pope was at the UN, he still said he didn't want to go in for family planning. It is a question of methods. Catholics aren't supposed to use artificial methods. But the natural methods (withdrawal, rhythm, etc) are highly unsuitable. Especially, in the developing countries, where there is no hygiene and no knowledge of any kind.

"It hasn't always been easy. There have been many times of discouragement. But I have been very fortunate. For better or for worse, I would live my life over again. When someone like me has been permitted to be a Mother Confessor to those who were in trouble, and has felt how important it was to be there, I ask you, can one expect anything better of one's life?

Doris Linder

Doris Linder is an American professor and historian who has recently completed a biography of Elise Ottesen-Jensen. On a visit to London in 1991, Ms Linder talked at length with me about Ottar and her rich life. I regret that more of Ms Linder's knowledge and insights cannot be included here. Her scholarly biography will be of great interest to those who wish to know more about Ottar. Here she tells the story of three Ottesen women's experiences with motherhood: Ottar's mother, her sister and Ottar herself.

"The television interview you quoted here has been very popular in Norway. It was shown in the 1970s to an enormous audience and in the 1980s, for the 25th anniversary of Norwegian television. So Ottar continues to be well-known. The only letters that Norwegian TV received in connection with the programme were from the area where she grew up and which she tells about in the interview, a region where pietistic viewpoints are common. It was a repeat of 100 years ago. They had the same observations to make: she was sinful to be so open about sexuality.

"Her parents had quite a different attitude from that of the region. Her father drank cognac; the children could dance around the Christmas tree; on Sundays they dared to laugh. It created quite a sensation when this 'brood' moved into the parsonage. Her mother had 18 children in all. The first five died promptly. The family was then living in the far north of Norway in a village that faced right out on the Arctic Sea. It is really grim country. Diphtheria and other contagious diseases were rampant. Her parents worked there as enthusiastic missionaries to the Lapps and fishermen. A sixth child survived while the couple lived there. There were to be six more. Elise was next to the last, the sister named Magnhild.

"Elise, in her late teens, was understudying a dentist in Stavanger, Norway in 1903. In the course of working with chemicals in the labouratory, there was an explosion that badly damaged her hands. She had to abandon the idea of being a dentist for, after months of operations, she lost three fingers and could not manipulate precise dental equipment.

"The tragedy of her sister's pregnancy out of wedlock soon added to a series of incidents which influenced her life and pushed her into new paths. When her father, Dean Ottesen, learned about the sister's situation he exploded in rage. There was nothing to do except send Magnhild abroad, otherwise this would disgrace the entire family. Magnhild was shipped off to Denmark in 1906. There were homes there to which she, a child of 16, could be sent during pregnancy. No information came from her parents; she was in disgrace. She was told nothing; all she knew is that after a beautiful experience with a boy neighbour, she had this emptiness inside her, of the child that was no more. Magnhild had to give away the child at birth. That's the way things were handled.

"Elise, who was undergoing operations on her maimed hands in another part of Norway, did not see Magnhild again until 1914 and did not yet perceive what a terrible impact the whole thing had on her younger sister. When Elise did see her and hear what happened she was shocked at what she had endured and by how much Magnhild talked about the little baby that was lost to her, of how she wondered what the child would look like. Magnhild had wanted to become a nurse. But because in her records it was stated that she had borne a child out of wedlock, she was barred from entering a nurses training programme. She could never do anything to earn her keep but work as a nurses aide. She deteriorated over the years. She was finally institutionalized in an asylum for the mentally disturbed in 1926. There she spent her time sewing baby clothes; she had a fixation about her loss. She died in 1934 at age 44.

"Elise also had a child out of wedlock. I am glad I can share this with you because I made such a point to find out about her child; there are endless errors in newspaper accounts about it so I copied the statement from the vital statistics. That 'a son was born to unwed Elise Ottesen and editor Albert Jensen in October 1917 and died two days later'. It was a sickly baby. Elise had puerperal fever that left her unable to bear children. She was terribly depressed after this for she had wanted a child. She and Albert finally did marry in 1931. But in 1935 when she came home from a lecture tour up north she found Albert in bed with a young girl who was staying with them. She was the daughter of a fellow syndicalist who lived in northern Sweden; her family had sent her to them so she could study music. Elise was terribly distraught and tried to figure out ways to salvage the marriage. It would take from spring 1935 until September 1937 for them to finally separate.

"It was in January 1936 that she was in an automobile

accident following a row. And it was Dr Luft who took care of her.

"Hers was a beautiful life. She overcame many personal challenges and was able to help so many people. That is what she wanted most to do."

Professor Rolf Luft

Of all who knew Mrs Ottesen-Jensen, Professor Rolf Luft was perhaps her closest friend. During World War II they resided in the same apartment building, and later they travelled together on medical missions. Professor Luft, an endocrinologist, was for many years the head of the Nobel Committee for Physiology and Medicine. I met him at his home one afternoon in 1990. He vowed to tell the truth about Ottar, saying, "Her real story is more interesting than the myths."

"I came into her life and she into mine in 1939, when I was on night duty at the hospital. I was called one night, somebody was very ill, in severe pain. I went to see. There was a Mrs Ottesen Jensen who had been in a car accident and who had concussion. She was the boss's private patient.

"That is the way I got to know her. I understood that she was in trouble; in fact this took place when her husband left her. This is the first time I've told this, but I'm old myself, so what the hell. To me it is more important, more human, more understandable to say that this was a woman with problems, who could channel her problems in a beautiful way. This will be more important to people who read this than to say she was born a giant. I said in one speech, 'She channelled her own adversities into something good for mankind.' It's so much easier to understand humans if you know what they went through.

"Her husband was a syndicalist, a union leader in Sweden, and was chief editor of the paper. He had been in jail many times for his beliefs. She worshipped him. And he left her for a young girl whom they had taken into their home. Ottar found them together, a typical little dramatic story. She left the house and that's when she had the car accident. I suppose people will detest me for telling this, but why not tell the truth? She was 51. After a while it quietened down and they became friends again. I got to know the husband and we often had dinner, the three of us – not the other woman although he eventually married her many years later.

"She had a son that died; he would have been my age. At

one point she was writing her memoirs and asked 'Do you want me to write about you?' I said 'No.' But we had a very special relationship, so she wrote, 'When I was sick he came into my room. I had had a son who died young, now I have another son.' You see, my real mother came from a very, very poor family of factory workers in the southern province. I never read a book in my childhood. I started to read on my own, and then I read everything, but was totally unintellectual. Ottar was the one that came into my life as a substitute; she took care of the other part of my life and she had an enormous impact on me. Through her I went into analysis; it helped me and I became a rather well-known national figure. And she was like a mother, jealous like hell on a couple of occasions.

"It's my belief that her emotional life with Albert Jensen was not very satisfactory. There must have been something missing. I think she had inhibitions, she had problems herself. A woman with sexual problems, perhaps, and one sign is, he left her for a young nobody with light blue-eyes and blonde hair.

"Every fifth year there was a big birthday party for her and I always gave a speech. There was one occasion when I said, 'All of us, all of you come to her so often with your problems, sitting at her feet, crying and she helps you, nobody ever asks if she has problems. None of you have ever asked her if she has problems. I know she has. And she has,' I said (I put it softly) 'I have the feeling that she has fooled us with the story of her sister, that there are other things that she has never disclosed to anybody.' When we got home that evening, she was furious. I had never seen her like that before or after. And she banged her fist on the table, 'You must promise me never ever to say anything like that about me or discuss it or anything.' I was flabbergasted, but then I understood. You see, I had touched a sore point.

"She was able to communicate an idea in a way that is acceptable and makes people feel that it isn't quite as serious as it might be. I remember once when she was going to talk to the cadets in the Air Force. I could just imagine what they were saying before she came. She began speaking and after a while they were just fascinated. The applause was enormous.

"When it came to her work, 'the cause', then she was tough, absolutely solid rock and she was so honest, that they couldn't pull her leg at all. She couldn't be humourous about herself. I haven't thought about it for a long time. There were, in fact two persons. When she was with me she could laugh and tell jokes. But when it came to the office of discussion of her organization, she was a rock. She was sharp like a knife, a completely different person.

"She had eccentric ideas perhaps, but people were devoted to her. She had an aura around her. For instance, long ago, before I married, this was a bachelor's apartment. Many people were coming and going here. When she came, she became the centrepiece within half an hour. There were journalists, actors, actresses, writers, doctors, scientists – but somehow she became the focus of interest and she liked it. Sometimes full of vanity, she said, 'Clothes don't mean a thing to me.' but she could stand for half an hour in front of the mirror trying on hats. Being a syndicalist money meant nothing to her, she left nothing when she died, she spent all the money, not very much on herself. She was a woman, but she didn't want people to see her real self; she played an act and she did it well.

"One story which is not known is that she was proposed for the Nobel Peace Prize. I think it was a Swedish Cabinet Minister and some other ministers who proposed it. She was then already on one of my wards with cancer – it was a terrible death, she had too much radium. Before the October it was announced, we were pretty sure that she would get it. We had planned that her niece's husband and I would escort her up the aisle and she would wear her doctor's hat. I promised her I'd keep her upright and she laughed. She said. 'Of course you know I am not at all interested in this, this is for the IPPF.'

"Then came the news that in that particular year they would not give anyone the prize. They postponed it to the next year. But Ottar wouldn't live that long. I had to go in and tell her. I was so furious, I could have gone to war against Norway. I think what happened was that Norway was not ready for it. Norway was a little backward and they were not ready for planned parenthood. It was a great tragedy. It would have been a great achievement and she deserved it. After that, she started to go downhill. She discussed her funeral with me and decided she didn't want a priest or a religious ceremony and so we decided that I would officiate.

"In Norwegian there is a saying 'It is better to have loved and suffered than never to have loved'. We recited that. That's her life: she had loved and she had suffered."

Elise Ottesen-Jensen

1886	Born Hoyland, Norway (17th of 18 children)
1905	Laboratory accident which resulted in the amputation of thumbs and a finger
1906	Sister Magnhild was banished to Denmark for pregnancy out of wedlock
1917	Gave birth (unwed) to a son who died two days later
1923	Delivered first public speech on family planning
1924	Learnt to place diaphragms, started travelling throughout Sweden
1931	Married Swedish union organizer Albert Jensen
1933	Created Swedish Association for Sex Education (RFSU)
1952	Founder member of the International Planned Parenthood Federation, Bombay
1973	Died (aged 87)
1986	Statue erected in her honour in Sandes, Norway

Chapter 4
Sylvia Fernando (1904–1983)

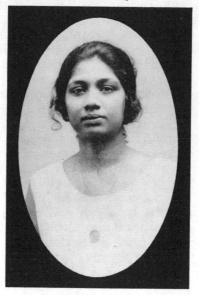

Sylvia Fernando, the founder of the Family Planning Association of Sri Lanka, shortly after her wedding. Circa 1934.

The house was open to all

The tropical island nation of Sri Lanka (formerly known as Ceylon) sits, tear-drop shape, off the south-eastern tip of India. The island's spices brought Arab, Dutch, Portuguese and, later, British conqueror-traders to its shores where many settled. Their ancestors have joined with the Sinhalese, originally from Northern India and with the Tamils from its south, to constitute the patchwork of ethnic and religious groups of modern Sri Lanka. The first census, held in 1871, counted two and a half million inhabitants. A century later, the population reached 13 million; today it stands at 17 million, becoming one the of most densely populated agricultural countries in the world.

Following Sri Lankan independence from Britain in 1948, its government quickly took note of its demographic expansion. At the Second World Health Assembly in 1949, the Sri Lankan Health Minister, who was later to become Prime Minister, S.W.R.D. Bandaranaike, warned the world community of the dangers of population growth.

Throughout the next decade, Sri Lanka's proposal to establish a Population Committee within the World Health Organization was opposed by those who insisted that it should not be a concern for an international body. Within Sri Lanka, however, the move to establish family planning services moved on, through the vision and determination of a small but dynamic group of volunteers led by a remarkable woman. Sylvia Fernando's courage and sensitivity resulted in one of the most successful family planning programmes in the world.

Sri Lanka is often cited as a nation which made excellent social policy decisions from independence onward. Universal education and health care were the cornerstones of its socio-economic development. Unfortunately, the resources on which these policies were to rely were the commodities tea, jute and rubber, which have suffered the volatility of world market prices. In addition, the issue of cultural and political autonomy for the Tamil population burst into rebellion in 1983. Since then Sri Lanka has been the scene of escalating violence, economic stagnation and increasing poverty.

When talking with those who knew Sylvia Fernando, the subject of her sensitivity to ethnic diversity was often raised. In the early 1950s when she commenced her effort to bring family planning to Ceylon, she skillfully gathered together a representative group of the island's peoples and religions before undertaking any initiatives. Her personal charm convinced politicians, volunteers, medical personnel, friends and family that planned parenthood was essential to the well-being of mother and child, the family and the nation.

Phyllis Dissanayake

The chosen successor of Sylvia Fernando, Phyllis Dissanayake, came to meet me at the offices of the Family Planning Association of Sri Lanka. Her affectionate description of her mentor was alternately humorous and melancholy.

"Mrs Fernando was first my teacher. When she finished her BA degree she got a job teaching the sixth form at Ladies College. I got to know her very well and we became friends. Sylvia's mother was a big influence on her, I'm sure. She was very keen on community service and was a prison visitor. Her father was a gynaecologist-obstetrician. He was Medical Superintendent of the De Sousa Maternity Hospital. I'm sure both parents were concerned about the health and welfare of families at the time, even though family planning was not yet known. Sylvia must have heard about all these problems as she was growing up.

"Her mother worked at the Dean's Road Clinic and the Social Service League and realized that every year the same women turned up pregnant. Before they could finish feeding one child they had another. As a result babies and mothers were very sickly. Sylvia saw for herself when she went with her mother that it was too many too soon. Sylvia's concern was for the health of the mother and child, not any economic theories about population; she wasn't thinking about the world at large.

"Sylvia was a friend of the president of the All Ceylon Women's Conference, an umbrella group of women's organizations. She used to help her a lot, go and work at her house and by means of that she also went to conferences abroad. There she met people who were discussing family planning abroad, people like Margaret Sanger, Dorothy Brush, Dr Clarence Gamble. At the time ships were the sole mode of transportation and if you were travelling in Asia, one of the ports visited was Colombo. So when these pioneers came to Sri Lanka, Sylvia would organize meetings with politicians or tea parties and dinners. She was very friendly with politicians and cabinet members who were friends of her husband or his school mates and family acquaintances. The age of democracy hadn't really come. It was people who had education and some money, people of standing, who were cabinet ministers. Sylvia had been in university with all these people. Mrs Bandaranaike (later to become Prime Minister of Sri Lanka on the death of her husband) was a volunteer in the FPA clinic; she took care of the patient card file. People who came into the limelight later were friends of Sylvia. Once she had the meeting at Major Jayawardene's house to which cabinet ministers came so that she could influence them and get support.

"At the time family planning was a dirty word; it was not something you talked about. Some declared that we were corrupting the morals of society in addition to interfering with peoples' very private affairs. Sex was a dirty word, especially among the Buddhist and Hindu population. When we received our first grant from government we had to promise to keep it secret, for they feared the political fall-out if it were made known. Even in the 1960s there were times when the propaganda officers held meetings and talked about family planning which resulted in buckets of dirt thrown at them because they were 'talking dirty things'. If 'God gave children', we shouldn't interfere. Ethnic and religious issues were factors as well. If people were looking for reasons to oppose family planning, they would say that the ethnic ratios would be altered. There were those who said that the Sinhalese were over two-thirds of the population and you couldn't make the two-thirds into a minority by family planning. Others said we weren't doing enough in Tamil areas or in Muslim areas. Even now this is brought up occasionally as an argument. That is why Mrs Fernando wanted to have such a mixed group of people to help her; they were from all the different communities: Tamil, Buddhist, Christian, Muslim.

"For a long time she kept after me to join the family planning association but I was then teaching and didn't want to undertake anything else. She was looking for someone whom she could train to succeed her. That was very far-seeing. She had been the General Secretary from 1953 on and there was never any thought that anyone else would ever be in her shoes. But she looked to the future and felt that the time would come when she couldn't do it any longer. I finally agreed and she assigned me to the propaganda section. That was 1968. She got me to do things with her so that when the association was incorporated in 1970, at the election which followed, she could stand down as General Secretary. She announced that I would replace her, saying she would be in the background to train me. She wanted to devote herself to the propaganda work being done and to work in the Estate sector.

"She believed we ought to train a younger group to take over from the people who were getting old – the volunteers who kept the books, who went to the clinics and distributed contraceptives. She said we have to find younger people, but it wasn't easy because it turned out that younger people were all working. The original clinics were started by Mrs Fernando through doctors she knew personally. They just did it free and their well baby clinics in the out-stations became family planning clinics as well. She trained them here and then they went back to their own areas.

"The first president of the FPA was Mrs Ratnam, a Canadian

woman doctor who was somewhat of an international figure. She had run a family planning clinic in 1937 here in her private medical practice. Sylvia was the General Secretary, the person who actually ran the association. She believed very strongly that the president should always be Sinhalese, Buddhist and a man. She felt that with a Christian at the head, there might be suspicions of undermining the Buddhists. She didn't want it said that the effort was anti-Sinhalese or anti-Buddhist. She also felt that women were still unable to command the degree of respect given a man. She probably was conservative in that way, but she was willing to run the organization and let someone else be the president, the visible leader.

"In the beginning, people who did this work encountered lots of barriers because they were considered as touching on the obscene, discussing matters that shouldn't be talked about. There was also a problem of male attitudes. Women would tell us not to write to them at home because their husband or mother-in-law would find out they are taking a contraceptive. It was especially true of Muslim women who, by the way, preferred the injection contraceptive because there was no trace; with the pill there was the risk of discovery.

"In 1965 when the government officially recognized family planning and took over, there were 85 clinics. They became part of the MCH [maternal and child health]. Then we began to concentrate on propaganda efforts. The age of leisured, elderly ladies with time to spare was coming to an end. It coincided with the realization that you couldn't run an association purely on volunteers because there had to be full-time workers with specialized skills. As the association grew, as the budget grew, we had to have people who knew about finance, and eventually, in 1974, a full time executive director."

Leela Basnayake

Leela Basnayake is a past president of the Family Planning Association of Sri Lanka (1977–1980) A small, fragile-appearing woman, she is now in her late seventies. She admitted being intimidated by an 'oral history', saying that details are so often forgotten with passing time. That said, her admiration for Sylvia Fernando had not diminished with the passing years.

"I first met Sylvia when we were both involved in the All Ceylon Women's Conference, an umbrella organization which grouped all the major women's and service organizations of the country for the purpose of learning from and helping each other. I was a member of the Buddhist women's organization which was one of its affiliates. The different groups shared experience and problems, many of which were due to population pressures. The teachers' association, for example, was talking about the number of children in classes, the lack of schools, etc. When we learned about the economic impact of the fast-growing population, we felt that something should be done. The health and financial problems of the mother and family were increasing everywhere.

"I remember vividly an incident that took place at the Dean's Road Clinic when I started working there. One was of a mother of eight, falling down at my feet, sobbing, 'Why were we not told of these things long ago? I have suffered in vain!' She was not only sad, she was angry that such valuable information had only been available to a privileged few. That was the first thing that prompted us to start the association and to work hard. There were some 14 or 15 of us who were the original locals who got interested in this.

"Sylvia was a very zealous person, always trying to make people join the association, work for it, saying, 'You can do it, why don't you try it?' She was one of the most dynamic people I've ever known, full of life, very persuasive, always laughing, with laughing eyes. She went to England on an All Ceylon Women's Conference and I think it was there that she met someone from Sweden, a Mrs Ottesen-Jensen. She came back full of enthusiasm. That is how she got into family planning.

"We never brought the subject of family planning into the All Ceylon Women's Conference because that would have been going too far. There were many Muslim, Buddhist and Hindu women. It would not have been acceptable. There was no sex education at the time. It was like the early Victorian days. Girls were supposed to be pure and ignorant. That was the criterion for marrying off a young daughter: she had to be thoroughly ignorant of the facts of life. They did not know how the human body functions. They did not know how conception took place. We had to explain from the very beginning.

"In the rural areas there were mixed schools so I think village girls were, in a way, more fortunate than us because we were separated in boys schools, girls schools. They could at least talk to each other. If we talked to a boy, some friend would report us to our mother who would get highly excited and report it to the father. To give you an example, our current medical director, Dr Dissanayake, started lecturing about a year ago, in 1990, on human sexuality. The place was terribly crowded. After the first lecture, the mothers came because they wanted to learn as well. So you can imagine what a lack of knowledge there is.

"We were considered vulgar and shameless people when we began our work in 1953. People thought family planning was something essentially for the family and certainly not to be discussed in public. There were letters to the editors written about family planning, about how even Buddhist ladies had taken this up and were involved in this scandalous affair. Letters from Catholic associations, from priests. At one point I was president of the Buddhist Women's Association. I used to receive horrible letters, saying either resign from the Family Planning Association or resign from the Buddhist Association. But I had great encouragement from my husband who helped me put up with it or throw the letters in the waste basket or burn them. So in that way I was able to carry on, otherwise it would have become a personal problem for me. I know from experience that you must have the assistance of your husband to be successful. If he is opposing you it would be very difficult.

Sylvia had no such trouble. Her husband, an electrical engineer, was very enthusiastic about family planning. When she got involved she was greatly served by her entire family: her mother, her aunt, her brother, daughter, husband – everybody. The whole family was involved. They all had the sense of social duty and service. Sylvia was a Christian and she, like all of us, did not believe in abortion. Some of our members were wondering if we should have abortion since we had so many people requesting them. Sylvia was quite adamant that the Family Planning Association have nothing to do with abortion. And we have kept that up to this very day. We advised the mothers to come to us soon after giving birth so we could instruct them about spacing the children.

"When the government programme began, all the government doctors were trained here. They would come and Sylvia would give them an introductory speech and then Dr Siva Chinnatamby would give them a medical talk. But the inspirational talk, the initiation of those doctors as to why and how they should be involved with family planing – that was given by Sylvia. She was a forthright person, she told them about the economics of the country, and since we were increasing in numbers she practically told them it was their duty to adopt these new methods of contraception, new ways of thinking. Her primary concern was family welfare in general. In those days we didn't talk about women's rights, that came later. We emphasized the economic situation of families, the demographic situation – that kind of thing. It was the duty of these young doctors to appreciate this. She would try to be very tactful but she was a direct sort of person. She did it with humour and kindness. When you heard her you wanted to get up and do something. It was almost like taking a vow."

Dr Siva Chinnatamby

I arrived at the home of Dr Siva Chinnatamby, where she has practised medicine for decades, on a quiet hot Sunday during monsoon season. She had asked me to come to her home because she was waiting for a call from a woman who was soon to go into labour. She wanted to be near the phone. We talked in her sitting room, a large room with a huge ceiling fan.

Following our talk, Dr Chinnatamby, who is a Tamil Sri Lankan, and a former President of the Asia Oceana Association of Gynaecologists and Obstetricians, took me into her office where I saw the photographs, diplomas and awards she has collected over the years.

As the medical advisor to the fledgling Family Planning Association, Dr Chinnatamby was instrumental in introducing new contraceptive methods to Sri Lanka. She, like many others even today, have been denounced for introducing modern methods from abroad.

"When I came back to Ceylon, following specialization in London, I worked in the De Sousa Hospital for Women. As a consultant in charge of the emergency cases, I had many cases admitted, day and night, for complications of child birth; haemorrhage, ruptured uterus, infection. Deliveries took place in the home and were assisted by untrained midwives. Complications were very high. I realized that 95 per cent of the women had more than 10 children and that these complications were preventable. One woman I cared for had 26 children. With the 26th baby she came to the hospital dying. She was 43 and had been married over 30 years, a baby every year.

"When Sylvia Fernando began her work to create the Family Planning Association she wanted to be sure to have good medical services and advice. She contacted my boss, Dr P.R. Thiagarajah, a gynaecologist with whom I had worked before I left for studies abroad. He said, 'Sylvia, there is someone coming back to Ceylon whom you must catch for your work.' She didn't know me but, through him, I went to talk to her and she said 'We would love to have you.' But I said, 'On one condition, I must be allowed to do sub-fertility because that is my speciality.' She replied, 'Oh yes, we will call it Mothers' Welfare Clinic. The idea is that every child is a wanted child. Not only the women who have too many children, but the others who want to have children.' So I became the medical consultant for the FPA. And in September 1953, we opened the very first clinic at the De Sousa Hospital for Women.

"At the first session we had about 32 women come. Almost all of them had more than five children. They came after it was announced in the paper. Thereafter it was spread by word of mouth and by home visitors also. Women did not tell their husbands that they were coming to the family planning clinic. They wouldn't even enter at the main entrance; they would come to the side entrance so as not to be recognized. They came, learned about the methods and promised to use them but actually not more than 5 per cent were using them at the end of the first year.

"We decided to send home visitors around to find out why the discontinuation was so high. At the sight of the visitors, doors were banged shut, windows were closed because mothers-in-law were in the house. When we were able, we asked the women personally, 'Why don't you like the mechanical devices, like the diaphragm. You learned to use it easily?' They replied, 'My husband doesn't like the smell of rubber'. Or 'We have no place to keep it out of the reach of children.' Or 'There's no place to wash it; we have a common tap with other families.' And 'After washing it I put it to dry and the crow took it away.' Men said the condom interfered with their sensation and they had no place of disposing of it after use because of the common lavatories. Everyone would know they were using them. So all this had to be faced. Progress was very, very slow.

"When I attended the IPPF Conference in New Delhi in 1959, I met Dr Pincus, the father of the pill. He presented a paper on the oral hormonal contraceptive. He had done the experiments, and the tests proved that progesterone given to women cyclically was reliable. I asked Dr Pincus if I could start a research project in Ceylon. He said 'Yes, but you had better come with me to America and see for yourself.' I was his house guest in Boston then went to Haiti and Puerto Rico. I'm glad I went because I found women of the same soci-economic class as ours using it contentedly, without any concern for side effects or anything. The pap smear was yet not known in Ceylon. So Dr Pincus agreed that I would send all the pap smears to the US saying, 'We will do the routine checkup of the acceptors so that they won't blame the pill if they develop cancer.'

"Progress was rather slow. There was a fear at that time that Western scientists were using women in developing countries as guinea pigs. I made it a point to emphasize that I asked for the pill; the pill was brought into this country at my request.

"The second method was the loop. Since the FPA didn't have sufficient room to accommodate the sterilization equipment, and examining tables, I started the IUD clinic here in my office at home. After two years time we had enough experience to report to the government committee who then approved the Lippes Loop for use here. Then came Depo-Provera. I heard about it through a project in Chiang Mai in Thailand. I went there to learn about it and came away very impressed. Women were queuing up, long queues, getting an injection in the arm and going away contented. But there were certain side-effects, absence of periods or a little spotting, etc. But the fact that it was used only once in 90 days was an attraction. I came back and asked for trials to be done and it was introduced in 1968. What was important was that every case, no matter what method was used, the pill, the loop, Depo-Provera, the women underwent a pap smear examination. I wanted to be 100 per cent sure. We did a few trials of women over 35, non-smokers, on the Pill and we did not regret that we were so cautious. Now they are in their sixties; they come for checkups and everything is normal, no cancers. Next we moved into the surgical methods, vasectomy and tubectomy the patient goes off after two hours.

"The latest method is Norplant, which was introduced here in 1985 by the Population Council and Family Health International. We were invited to go to Indonesia to view the project there. We introduced Norplant five years ago; people have accepted it. It is a very reliable method and the important thing is that fertility returns after a couple of months, so it is a very popular method. [Norplant is a slow-release hormonal contraceptive device, surgically implanted beneath the skin of the arm.] The only problem is that it is very expensive. Here someone has to sponsor the costs. And we must train all the doctors. You can't do it without good training, not just insertion, but removal as well. And of course you need a good referral system in case the woman has questions she wants answered.

"Five or six years ago I had a lot of problems with letters to the Editor; there were at least 10 or more letters asking, for example, 'Why is Depo-Provera not used in America when it is used in Sri Lanka. Are our women guinea pigs?' I wrote a centre page article in the *Daily News* giving the pros and cons, what research evidence was available; I quoted many countries using it, saying that we had done a very strict observation of the cases, total examinations done from breasts to the gynaecological and not a single problem case. That put a stop to it. Those letters were sometimes depressing, personally. Since I am from a minority ethnic group, they say I want to decimate the Sinhalese population, for example. That was sad, very ugly. But people who knew me, because I had a bigger practice among the Sinhalese than among the Tamils, said, 'Carry on, don't bother about all this..' That gave me the moral support to face it – so that it wasn't so personal. Of course Sylvia Fernando gave me a lot of encouragement. She was like a mother, saying 'Don't let them bother you, dear'. She gave moral support, and that was very important for me.

"I was the youngest of five children. My elder sister died of viral fever three months after delivery of her first child. My second sister married fairly young, at 19 I believe, when I was about six years old. She died also, 10 days after childbirth from pulmonary embolism, clots in the lungs. I was determined to contribute to the reduction of maternal and child mortality. I believe a home without a mother is like a house without a light, and that every child should be a wanted child. I never married. I could have easily married; there were a couple of individuals who expressed interest in me but my career came first. Sometimes, for example, with a bad case I didn't get home for three days, working day and night. So if I had a family of my own, it would have been difficult, to say the least.

"The main thing is that I was interested in my work. It involved me completely, saving so many lives, or trying my best. And the job satisfaction of my work in infertility was immense. There are still a great many illegal abortions in Sri Lanka. One gynaecologist told me he sees 20 a day in his hospital service. It will never be legal here, it is too controversial for government to get involved.

"I enjoyed working with Sylvia Fernando. She encouraged me to do whatever I wanted and she stood by me if there was any criticism in the Council. She was a dynamic being. A very loveable person, very simple, articulate. She had fixed ideas; you couldn't budge her, shake her. One day her daughter, Nimali, called me and said, 'We must take mother to the hospital right away'. We rushed her there and while we were waiting for her room to be ready she passed away in my arms."

Nimali Kannangara

The daughter of Sylvia Fernando lives high in the hills of southern Sri Lanka, among tea and rubber estates. A former director of Save the Children in Sri Lanka, Nimali Kannangara now resides and works at St Joseph's Convent in Deniyaya. The drive to visit her took place during Vesak, the annual Buddhist holiday. Throughout the journey each village, decorated and filled with festival goers, was hosting a parade, a musical event, a ceremony of some sort. In the quiet of her sitting room, overlooking distant hills, Mrs Kannangara, gave some personal insights into her mothers' character and motivations.

"Both my grandmother and mother were extraordinary individuals. The society at the time was very British. My grandmother, for example, was married in a frock, with a hat. There was an active decision among minorities within the Tamil and Sinhalese population to work with the colonial authorities. And in working with them, recreated British society. They dressed in European clothes, went to the races; most of them couldn't speak Sinhala. It was in that context that my grandmother – my grandfather was an obstetrician who saw over and again the poverty around them – worked for the common good, a sort of *noblesse oblige* of the times.

"After her degree mother did research in sociology and became very knowledgeable about caste. She worked with several foreign sociologists, among whom were Bryce Ryand and Edmond Leach who were looking at caste. Every student who came within several hundred miles of her was sent to consult her. She would help them set up their research project in some village and counsel them. She worked with these sociologists who came to consult her right to the end of her life. The fact that she took pains to understand the caste system and find value in it as well as flaws was, I think, an expression of her interest in people. Her work in sociology fascinated her; it was her light relief, I think. She enjoyed using her brain, her intellect. I don't know if family planning required her to use her intellect, mostly just her personality and organizational skills.

"Mother was one of the earliest modern women I have known, but in her relationship with her husband she was traditional. She was one of the first, if not the very first, woman to have a driver's license. My father was never ever driven by her. It was too traumatic because she would drive in the middle of the road, very slowly. And when she backed up she would get someone else to look. She drove me everywhere – was the chauffeur for school – always talking and not looking at the road. She parked in the nearest spot to where she was going, regardless of the fact that it might be an official parking place, reserved for the municipal commissioners or some such. She was so charming to the policeman who turned up, that everything was forgiven. That was the way she handled everything: she just did it.

"When she started building the family planning office building, my father calculated its costs – with his hair standing on end. She had only one third of the money and no official permission from Government. But over dinner she had made the Prime Minister or somebody say that he would give her the land. And she started in. My father was very proud of her. He used to have to do the accounts for the Association and would say, 'What's this nonsense I have so much work to do'. But he did it like a lamb.

"She had confidence – a quite dangerous confidence – that people spoke the truth when they told her something, and that logic is obvious to everyone. She believed in things like loyalty, and she suffered a great deal for it. If she thought something was logical for her, then it must be for others. If it was best for a woman to space her children, surely everybody would recognize it sooner or later. It was almost a touch of naïvete.

"She was a religious woman, certainly more than most. She was an active Protestant. She recognized that she was in a fortunate situation and wanted to say thank you to God. This was a powerful feature of her character. Service to those less fortunate was very much a part of our lives because we were so fortunate. People who stayed at our house – foreign researchers, visiting family planners, our school chums – were always struck by the fact that no matter how busy my parents were – and my father, too, was frightfully busy – they would spend a time together, alone, each evening, chatting and chuckling about the days events. And then they would say their prayers.

"There wasn't an ounce of personal ambition in her. If one understands that, her leadership style becomes clearer. I remember how she talked to politicians at dinner and how she convinced them that they had thought up the idea first. That's how she got things to happen. Always pleasantly, charmingly. Our house was the FPA office for all the years it didn't exist elsewhere. Our friends came to the house after school, or sports. We'd always be falling over visiting family planners or researchers. But we knew we had just as much right as anybody else to bring our friends home. Her outside interests did not mean rejection of us. We children used to have to turn envelopes. The FPA couldn't afford to buy envelopes, so my classmates and I would come home for lunch and be given enormous stacks of old envelopes. For hours, we turned enveloped for the FPA correspondence. We were bribed with lunch and ice-cream. Were we ever told what the envelopes were needed for? I don't think we were. I don't think she did explain family planning to me ever. We just absorbed it from listening in and living with her.

"I realize that she always feared that family planning would be another minority struggle. She anticipated that minority anxieties would surface sooner or later. A few people realized – and my mother was one of them – that as the population grew and resources had to be spread thinner and thinner, minority questions would surface and no way was she going to allow the family planning association to be caught in that at all. The walls of our garden were labelled with insults. Anonymous callers, dreadful letters. The whole thing ranging from calling her 'a traitor to the Singhala race', because she was helping to decimate the Singhalese and increase the number of Tamils. The Catholics said she was violating God's law. The Buddhists declared that family planning interferes with Nature's laws and upsets the karmic cycle.

One day a delegation of Buddhist priests came to the house. My father and I were petrified. But mother was very interested. They said, 'Do you realize the evil you are doing? You will have to live 750 lives in the future to expiate this sin.' Mother was ready to settle down for a nice chat. But then she forgot herself and sat on a chair. Our servant had to scuffle up and pull her off and put white cloths on the chairs so they could sit on them. But mother found it all very interesting and not alarming at all.

"You see, my grandmother did charitable work but I think mother moved away from that in her thinking and beliefs. She realized that improvement of the condition of women or family planning could not be done as an act of charity. It had to be much more democratic, depending on fundamental skills and capabilities. Working in the estates reinforced my mothers notion that family planning is just the beginning for women; they must have income, be helped to control their lives. She believed strongly that you had to provide information and access, not food and clothing, handouts, but enabling information and access, enhancing women's capabilities. She got to know Lady Rama Rau long before she became eminent in the Indian family planning movement. She would come and spend weeks here; they would talk for hours at a time. Mother would help her write up ideas and then they would send them off to await a reply anxiously.

"Mother always had the fear that methods of contraception hadn't been tested enough, or looked at enough. There were few longitudinal studies available and she always remained scep- tical, especially when pharmaceutical firms began to contact the Family Planning Association offering money for research or trials. She may have worried about how to raise money for the roof of the FPA building but she wouldn't allow it to be obtained through those commercial means. She didn't want anything to do with them. She was not going to let them turn us into a laboratory.

"It was very difficult to have something to do with her and remain selfish. She was completely devoid of person ambition. She was constantly sending off the young people to conferences instead of going herself, constantly pushing them forward. At 79 when she died, she still had hordes of people coming to talk with her. I think there were several things which she found difficult to accept – new trends and new techniques. Do you remember my story about the envelopes, how we had so little money that we had to fold them ourselves. Well, mother asked for a telephone number once and was given it on a large piece of paper with the family planning address printed on top. The discrepancy between the days when they didn't have money to buy envelopes and then using a whole sheet of creamy white paper to write a telephone number – she thought about it a lot. She was never cynical enough to take all that sort of thing and the corruption of motive in her stride. Now we take it for granted that the bigger the institution the less spiritually motivated (the more corrupt) it is likely to be, the higher the costs versus benefits. She was unprepared for that and I think her last years were discoloured by it.

"I think she was always surprised at the things that were said. The things she found painful were instances where you would be compromised or the profit-motive reared its head. She never could understand that it was almost inevitable, when there was a lot of money involved, jobs and perks to be had. Each sign of this was a fresh blow to her, almost as bad as the first blow.

When she died my father and I received over one thousand letters, one thousand, from people we didn't know."

Sylvia Fernando

1904	Born Colombo, Ceylon
	Studied sociology and economics, University of Colombo
1930	Married Fernando, an engineer
1946	Visit to Sweden: obtained funding for pilot Family Planning Association Programme
1948	Independence of Ceylon/Sri Lanka
1953	Created Family Planning Association of Sri Lanka
	Opened Regional Office of IPPF in Colombo
1965	Government commenced National Family Planning Programme
1983	Died in Colombo

Chapter 5
Constance Goh Kok Kee
(b. 1906)

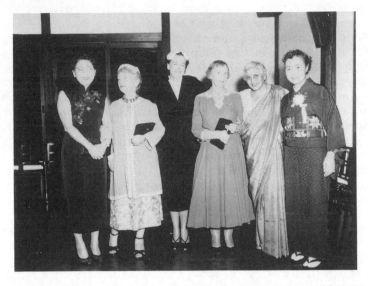

*From left to right: Constance Goh Kok Kee (Singapore), Margaret
Sanger (USA), Elizabeth M. Jolly (Hong Kong), Elise Ottesen-Jensen
(Sweden), Lady Rama Rau (India), Senator Shidzue Kato (Japan)
at the 5th International Conference on Planned Parenthood,
Tokyo, 1955.*

Suffering has been my life long concern

When Sir Stamford Raffles of the British East India Company
was searching for a trading centre on the rich Malay peninsula,
the deep-water harbour of Singapore offered optimum facilities.
In 1819 Singapore was established as a shipping centre for tin
and rubber and by 1924 was ceded to Britain, to be administered by the Governor General of India. During the Second
World War, the city was a prize catch for Japanese forces
who sought to control the people, commerce and resources of
south-east Asia. The first Japanese bombs fell on Singapore,

at the same time as their bombs fell on Pearl Harbor, Hawaii, 7 December 1941. The city remained under Japanese control for the next three and a half years, until August 1945.

It was because of the conditions she witnessed during and after the war that Constance Goh Kok Kee became an active promoter of planned parenthood. By 1949, the small group of volunteers working with Mrs Goh had formed the Family Planning Association of Singapore (renamed the Singapore Planned Parenthood Association in 1986), which delivered its services from her husband's office.

For the next 17 years, the association was the only organized agency delivering family planning services to the people of Singapore. As one of the earliest associations in Asia, it was a founder member of the International Planned Parenthood Federation (IPPF) in 1952. Through the work of the association, Mrs Goh and her colleagues began to enlist the support of government officials and politicians. When in 1963 she organized an IPPF conference in Singapore she was careful to invite the Prime Minister Lee Kuan Yew to officially open the meeting. His presence gave much needed status and impetus to the family planning movement locally and regionally.

In 1960, the population of the city which Constance Goh jokingly says is one seventh the size of Long Island, New York, at low tide, was 1.634 million. The growth rate stood at 4.6 per cent.[1] Today Singaporeans number 2.8 million and the growth rate has decreased to 1.3 per cent.[2] This remarkable reduction in growth rate is due largely to the effective family planning programme created by the government of Singapore in 1966. It has been so effective that it has now come under scrutiny. Indeed, former Prime Minister Lee recently criticized young women of the tiny island nation, saying that they were too well educated and not interested enough in having children. Dr Paul Cheung, director of the Ministry of Health's Population Planning Unit, is quoted as saying that the task now is to persuade 'reluctant' Singaporean couples who can afford it to have more children.[3]

Mrs Constance Goh Kok Kee

Mrs Goh, the pioneer of family planning in Singapore, is now in her 86th year. She was waiting for me in the upstairs sitting room of her home. Dressed in trousers and a flowered shirt, her greeting was informal, her laughter deep and rich. For the occasion she had prepared tea, a special cake and had ready documents she felt would be of interest. Her language showed a strong Christian faith; she expressed deep concern about the state of the world. We talked first of her childhood and her background as a Chinese Singaporean.

"We lived in Xiamen (Amoy), in the southern part of China, a night's trip from Hong Kong and across the straits from Taiwan. The big family house, called a *yahmen*, was shared with uncles and many relatives. I was number six in a row of girls. I was the first child of my parents but number six in the family. Because I was a girl I was neglected and often sick. Two years after my birth, a boy was born to an uncle so the family finally had a male. In large Oriental households, the daughters-in-law were treated as upper servants. There were many servants to supervise and that was my mother's duty, to supervise a host of servants.

"We were Presbyterian. The grandfather on my father's side was an elder and he was a judge at the same time. That was very rare in those days because Christians were not put in responsible positions, but grandfather succeeded. We were supposedly fairly well off. I had a personal nurse. She even went to school and sat next to me in the early days. My grandfather on my mother's side was a Presbyterian minister. His church is still in Amoy. One of these days I might be able to do something for that church but it is not functioning well now because the churches are forbidden to be too active.

"It was a big family and I seldom saw my father because he was in a different city, taking care of the family business. He came home three times a year: Chinese New Year, grandfather's birthday, grandmother's birthday. The result was that he and mother never had much to do with each other. Naturally he kept other women, and trouble with the concubines led mother to accept a job here in Singapore. That was 1918. She taught at the Chong Hock Chinese Girls' School at 21 Stanley Street. The school is still there, still a fine school.

"I finished schooling in 1924. I was then sent back to China, to Shanghai Baptist College, but my Chinese was not good enough for me to graduate. The Singapore standard of Chinese is quite different. In China, I had to know classical Chinese; it is an impossible language to learn – and to me it's useless. I would have had to take examinations in classical Chinese. I knew I couldn't, so I was allowed to choose what topics I wanted to study. The people there were very good to me. I took up the social sciences. I even took one course in astronomy and two in geology. Can you imagine? It was out of curiosity. In the

Christian ethics course they assigned a book entitled *Ecce Homo*. The theme of the book was 'Enthusiasm for Humanity' and this got stuck in my mind: *I* was going to be enthusiastic for humanity. I read the book when I was twenty years old and that saying became my guiding star.

"When you took the sociology courses, part of the course work entailed visiting prisons and courts, factories and farmers' homes. I was very upset by what I saw. In one factory girls, eight to 12 years old, were doing fine embroidery work in dimly-lit rooms. They were made to stand because if they sat down they would go to sleep. There were children less than eight years old, sitting around tubs of warm water, with silk worm cocoons floating on the water, to loosen the threads. The children were unravelling the threads day in and day out and many times they would be so tired, their heads would drop forward into the water.

"Seeing these things distressed me profoundly. Another incident that greatly impressed me was one involving my own family. The elders had decided that there should be a fish pond near my grandfather's grave. The workers who were to build the pond came from a nearby village. There was no heavy machinery in those days. They had poles with a disk on the end to pound the earth to make it hard. These young people worked all day, not for pay, they worked to earn *one meal*. I wondered, 'Had there been no grave to work on, what would they eat?'

"After two and a half years of study in Shanghai I came back to Singapore in 1930. I attended teachers' training school for my final year and then taught school for a year until I married. My husband was a public-health doctor. He was trained in Singapore, then went to England where he obtained a Diploma of Public Health and of Tropical Medicine. We met in Church in Singapore when he was in medical school. We had two children. A son who is a lawyer, and a daughter who passed away after only nine months of marriage. She was a musician. We built a church in her name. It is called Faith Methodist Church. By my son I have three wonderful grandchildren.

"We were fortunate to be able to remain together as a family all during the war. My husband had to work as a public-health doctor for the Japanese; he took care of the prisons, the police. We were lucky because a brother-in-law was the manager of the Overseas Chinese Bank which had a big office building in town. On the roof of the bank there was a club for business-men, a luncheon club. When the Japanese insisted that my brother-in-law keep the bank open he said, 'Only if I can have my family here with me.' So we were able to stay there with him as part of his family. For three and a half years we lived on the fifth floor of the Overseas Chinese Bank. It was a great big place with only partitions separating us. The first few nights we slept on the dining tables. It was so high up, no Japanese could get up. Since there was no electricity, there were no lifts. Every day my husband had to walk down 120 steps and walk up 120 steps so he refused to come home for lunch. He said he would be hungry all over again by the time he got to the office. We were very fortunate to be there. We survived on common sense. If there was no meat, we could eat bean curds. But many people with less money – the salaries were cut in half and the prices were tripled – were malnourished.

"It was after the war that we thought of the question of family planning. Seeing the distress and deplorable living conditions in Chinatown after the war led caring people to find ways and means to help. Children were running wild; if parents could not feed those they already had, how could they add more to the family? I started the first feeding centre for children in a converted motorshed in Havelock Road. The government gave the food, huge pots of rice, vegetables, fruit and some protein. It was cooked in the General Hospital and delivered to the centre. All we had to do was to organize the children. They were like wild animals. They were not orphans, they had families in Chinatown, but they had nothing to eat. By the time we ended the feeding programme there were 32 feeding centres all over Singapore. I had a team of helpers, most of them were foreigners. It was easy to get Europeans to serve because they have a tradition of service. I am sad to say that oriental people have never done too much for the public so it is not in their traditions. Nowadays there is more service but many still prefer to play mahjong or go to a fashion show or the hairdresser. I had a team of six or eight European women who came every day to help care for the children. They were so dirty, we had to scrub them.

"One day two brothers, eight and 10 years old, arrived covered with scabies. I didn't dare take them in my little car so I got two rickshaws. I dare not sit in a rickshaw with them; I took one rickshaw and the boys, the other. We went to the General Hospital Outpatient service and queued up with everyone else. Looking at the boys in disgust, the nurse turned to me and asked, 'Yours?' 'Yes', I replied. She could have killed me with her looks, but I replied yes because I wanted them to get attention quickly. The work was taxing. One day we counted some 360 children. Everyday after the feeding tasks I would take my helpers to a coffee shop and treat them to coffee and a cake. We would go home, take a shower and go straight to bed.

"We started classes in crafts which would make the children employable. We taught the girls to sew, book-binding for the boys. The little ones learned to play. The government was very pleased with my work. In 1951 or 52 they gave me the MBE. By King George, not the Queen. Before that they made me a JP in 1949. Before getting involved with family planning I was working with the YWCA and the Church. We ran night classes for girls. I was always concerned for girls – I don't care a hoot for the boys. It is the woman who carries the burden of childbearing; they worry about the family. More should be done for women on the grassroots level. Small-scale efforts to improve technology, to ease the burdens of women: bamboo pipes, improved stoves – little things.

"Family planning was proposed to allow women to space and limit the size of their families. It was seeing all the poverty of those post-war months that convinced us that something had to be done about family planning. We did not start willy-nilly, however. Recognizing our ignorance and inexperience, we sought advice from the University, the medical, legal, welfare and other professions and religious authorities. Public meetings were held and an MCH [maternal and child health] doctor, a social worker and a missionary were invited to speak. It resulted in the formation of an association to help these mothers. By far our greatest fear was the possible active opposition of religious bodies. To safeguard ourselves, a small committee was assigned to look into the teachings of the Bible, the Koran and the Hindu and Buddhist scriptures in regard to family planning.

"Fortunately there was nothing specific against our immediate objectives. Only the Roman Catholic Church voiced their opposition, saying family planning was against God and nature, and thus immoral. Roman Catholic nurses were forbidden to work in our clinics. The Catholic Church used to send me to hell twice a month. My friends told me that the priest regularly condemned me to hell for my work in family planning. Publicly!

"In June 1949, the Singapore Family Planning Association was officially inaugurated. At that time, our group had no knowledge or experience but we wrote to friends abroad and, using what little know-how we had personally, we plunged in. We sent voluntary workers around to spread the news. We sent social workers, church bible women – in those days there were bible women who went around urging people to come to church – so we used them to get the news to the community that there was a family planning clinic. On the last Friday of November we opened the first clinic in my husband's office in South Bridge Road. My husband was a devoted family man. He supported me in this work and offered his clinic. We worked there until we were able to move to other quarters. He didn't mind that I was condemned by the Church!

"On that first day there were six or seven of us and only one patient. Then the numbers increased quickly. The news spread by word of mouth. Few women could read. And we dared not say too much; we never had any publicity because if it was known we would be accused of trying to thrust something at other women, having nothing to do, or trying to get jobs. That was the attitude of the men, the public. So we worked quietly undercover. It caught on gradually. We wanted to create the climate for government to accept us, for people to think that we were doing good things for others. It was not that the Colonial Government was unaware of high birth rate problems but the Administration was loath to interfere in what it considered as the customs and habits of the governed people. At the time, Singapore had people from many different origins. We had nurses who could speak 11 different languages or dialects among them.

"As contraceptives, we used the cap and paste. It was very messy, troublesome, very expensive. I went to England one time to bargain with London Rubber. I talked to the manager, a Mr Reed, and said, 'The welfare of the people in the East is in your hands.' He reduced the price of the Dutch pessary from 3 dollars to 3 shillings; he halved the price. I still remember him.

"It was very difficult to persuade men to use condoms. Most men thought only of their own pleasure. They thought their fun might be spoiled, their health injured. The worship of ancestors influenced their attitudes as well. You must have sons to provide for you in the after-life and to carry on the family name, to serve you. The daughters get married and go away. It is the sons who remain and if you don't have sons you must try again and again. Many times their wives had to come to us in secret.

"One great boost came in 1951–52, a year or so after we started. Mr J.D.M. Smith, then the Colonial Treasurer, of his own volition allocated $5,000 for the association from the Colonial Treasury. The money was useful, to be sure, but more importantly, we could say, 'The Government presented us with money.' We could be open about our work at last. All of a sudden we were respectable, approved by government. I remember with affection and deep appreciation the boost he gave us.

"We had started the family planning association in 1949 and by 1952 we were a going concern with much to contribute. As such we were invited to the meeting at which IPPF was founded. We took our literature, our leaflets, drawings. And while we were going to receptions and all, Mrs Butcher was teaching a class of nurses on procedures, case cards. Our case card file was so wonderful it was copied by many other associations. We had a column how many children born, how many boys, girls, how many survivors. And we had a special column: how many children given away.

"We enjoyed our work. There was something about working together, a group of dedicated people – it was a wonderful fellowship, especially Lady and Sir Percy McNeice. Sir Percy was the City President. He was the first top civil servant to dare to associate himself with such a seemingly suspect organization as ours. It was said that some of his colleagues warned him about his job being at risk, but he became President of the Family Planning Association and remained with it for 10 years until his retirement. The value of his involvement and that of Lady McNeice's family was incalculable. They were on the top of the social scale and would give parties as fund raisers for us. I've since worked out thirty-four ways to make money! Small little efforts. People are such snobs, you know. They love to go to see the big houses to be able to say. 'I've been there'. We did that almost every month. For one dollar per person the hostess would provide a tea and a speaker on how to take care of your skin or how to lose weight... Everybody would pay a dollar and we would find ourselves with $200 for the family planning association.

"In 1963 we held a conference which was addressed by Prime Minister Lee. He came out clearly for family planning in Singapore. He was a very up and coming man and he could sense the future problems. He talked scientifically about the population pyramid; he was very good. We were very happy to have him at the conference. After he gave that speech, the Roman Catholic Church dare not say a word about family planning. They stopped sending m'e to hell. That's why I'm still here. Before that the Catholic Church refused to let their communicants work in the family planning clinics but after the Prime Minister made family planning a government policy, the Church shut up. I don't believe the Church will ever come to a better understanding of family planning. Their opposition is too deeply rooted. It is for us women to rebel. Catholicism is the same as communism: control from above. And worse yet, they say it is all in the name of God. They want to control the family – Pay, Pray and Obey. We must have a sense of urgency about all this. We are not *keen* enough. The politicians just pass the buck. They say it is the responsibility of the church, responsibility of the medical profession, responsibility of private organizations – just passing the buck. We should have universal involvement – of all sectors of society.

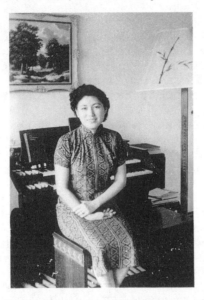

Constance Goh Kok Kee, founder of the Singapore Family Planning Association, in 1954.

"The early evolution and development of family planning activity in neighbouring areas occurred almost spontaneously, in tandem with the Singapore FPA. Our newspaper *The Straits Times*, was common to Malaya as well as Singapore and soon after the Association was formed, letters from individuals seeking advice started to arrive from all over the peninsula. Wherever possible they were put in touch with doctors or nurses who could help them, otherwise information and supplies were sent by mail. Volunteers visited Malaya, Sabah, Sarawak and Brunei and through their personal contacts, interested individuals started clinics with supplies provided through the Singapore FPA. In Sarawak we got the hospitals interested, we worked through the doctors and administrators. I travelled with very good friends, the Methodist bishop and his wife. That is also how I got to go to Burma as well, for in those days it was more difficult to go to Burma than to get to heaven. They took me along as a secretary and I contacted people at hospitals. I found a doctor who was willing to take our literature and give it out, but that was about all we were able to do. Nothing came out of it. The missionaries were very supportive; they knew the suffering of the people.

"In the past 40 years population in this region has multiplied several times, out-stripping resources to support them adequately. We started working in family planning over forty years ago and it seems to me that things are even worse now than when we first started. There are so many more people to motivate. And you need to motivate every one every day in their reproductive years.

"The family planning movement is top-heavy now, a lot of bureaucracy and waste. It's not for me to criticize, but so many meetings! For what? Bureaucracy is a waste. There is room for a lot of improvement, more zeal, more commitment. My experience shows that women started the family planning movement at the ground level and then when it became respectable the men jumped in. We need more women at all levels and especially up the hierarchy.

"On all of us weighs the heavy responsibility to help avert the future suffering of innocent lives."

Ethel Bloom

Constance Goh wrote to me, shortly after I returned to London and suggested that I contact one of her friends, a woman with whom she has kept up a correspondence and friendship since they met as young wives of medical doctors stationed in Malaysia just before the outbreak of the Second World War. An American, Ethel (Freddy) Bloom was captured and interned in a Japanese prisoner of war camp where she spent three and one half years. She was then a journalist and has since become an author and lecturer on teaching children with hearing impairments. When I wrote to ask if she would be willing to see me, I received a phone call saying: "Please come, anything to do with Sai Poh (the name by which Constance Goh is known to friends) fascinates and interests me." We met at her flat on a sunny London afternoon in 1991.

"It is impossible now to imagine what the attitude towards sex was in 1939 when I first met Constance. I was married to a doctor in the Indian medical service. His regiment was posted from India to Penang (Malaysia) when hostilities were threatened in Europe. I had been in India only a comparatively short time having come from New York via Dublin. I was still very American, in my early twenties, and was thrilled to be in Penang. I wanted to meet the people there. I didn't want to meet more Europeans; I knew them. I was anxious to meet some of the local people. Everybody thought this was a very odd attitude. I found myself involved with the YWCA, which isn't really my line of activity at all. I'm a journalist and writer. But it was the only way I could meet what some of my colleagues called 'black beetles'.

"One of the first 'black beetles' I met was Sai Poh who was married to Kok Kee, a doctor. It is hard to imagine it now, but at that time Kok Kee, who had been a King's Scholar at Cambridge, an outstanding doctor, was earning one third the salary of the European doctors in the same service. And often the Europeans were less qualified. Sai Poh was like a breath of fresh air. She wasn't one of these dainty, lovely, Chinese ladies. She wasn't pretty but had the most lovable face, enormous energy and was completely unafraid. She had been educated by the Methodists which meant that she was extremely literate and well-educated. It gave her a certain authority which less educated Chinese wives did not have and didn't even know about.

When she got interested in family planning? I don't know. But Sai Poh, due to her Methodist background, always knew what was right and what was wrong. When something was right, she would fight for it. Here we were in Penang with all the social strata and with this incredible attitude, which we now call prudery. It was simply the attitude that existed then, certain things were *not* discussed. We were not exactly Victorians and there was a certain amount of sleeping around, but it was always with enormous discretion and never discussed in detail. And here was Sai Poh, absolutely outspoken, absolutely determined that large families were bad for mothers, who were unhealthy due to frequent pregnancies; bad for the children because there were too many of them and not enough money to go around. The mortality rate was very high among children and mothers. So Sai Poh had to do something about it. I don't think she was doing anything about it in Penang, certainly not through the YWCA, but she had that attitude. She had a sense of social rightness.

"You must remember also the attitude which existed among the Chinese, among all the Asian families, where having lots of children was wealth and old-age care and anything that anybody wanted. Also, I suppose, most of the population was so poor that the only manhood that could be displayed was the size of the family. Even before Sai Poh put on her uniform and went to war, so-to-speak, she had this wonderfully outspoken, unafraid attitude which floored people because they didn't know what to make of it.

"Years later, when the King was to award her an MBE, I drove her to Buckingham Palace. But just before we were to leave, we discovered that she didn't have white gloves. On the way to the palace we stopped at Harrods and bought the white gloves. At the time the Communists were still a menace in her part of the world and people were concerned that they might have to leave their homes quickly at some point. Constance thought that jewellery was a good investment and could be taken easily if she had to flee. As we walked out of Harrod's we went through the jewellery department which had antique, as well as new, jewellery. There in the case was a very attractive plain bracelet of diamonds and emeralds. I can't remember the price, but say it was one thousand pounds. Sai Poh looked at the sales clerk and said, 'I'll give you five hundred'. Now this is Harrods. I thought, 'Sai Poh, one doesn't do this. . .' But the clerk just looked at her and said, 'Seven-fifty'. She bought it and wore it to the palace. Again, it was just Sai Poh being Sai Poh. Totally unselfconscious.

"If Constance was unafraid, it was because she had learned to stand up for herself; she just didn't care what people said or did if she knew she was right. I think she had a difficult time as a young bride in her husband's family home. His sisters gave her a really difficult time and I suspect anyone who could stand up to his sisters could stand up to anything. She and her husband had an unusual relationship. He certainly wasn't the type of husband who said you must be a nice little housewife. She ran his home; she brought up his children; she had complete freedom and was utterly emancipated.

"Our friendship was cemented when my first husband died very suddenly in Penang at age 27. It was a stupid death caused by poorly diagnosed pleurisy. I didn't know what to do. The war had started in Europe and if I returned to the US I would be able to take only one hundred pounds. I decided to get myself a job in Singapore. Constance dropped everything. She went down to Singapore ahead of me and told her friends and relatives to look after me. That's friendship for you. I was hired by a newspaper and living in Singapore was made a lot easier by the very fact that I was a friend of Constance. A year later, before Singapore fell, the newspaper was bombed. The military nurses left and others were needed, no matter how rotten they were. So I became a nurse.

"I remarried. Just nine days before Singapore fell to the Japanese, I married a doctor with whom I worked. We were interned for the remainder of the war, he in the military camp, I in the civilian camp. Sai Poh was delightful, she sent things in to me over and over again. When the Japanese finally capitulated, before we were sent back on troop ships, Philip and I went to see her. She brought out a little sandalwood chest full of old British money. The Japanese had saturated the country with what was known as banana dollars. They were useless. And she had real money. She opened the chest and said, 'Take what you want'. We had nothing so we took a bit, enough to get us to where we were going in England. That was Sai Poh, the friend who foresaw our needs."

Constance Goh Kok Kee

1906	Born Xiamen, China
1918	Moved to Singapore with mother
1924	Attended Shanghai Baptist College, studied sociology
1945	Created first children's feeding centre in post-war Singapore
1949	Initiated first voluntary family planning services in husband's office
1951	Made an MBE
1952	Singapore founder member of International Planned Parenthood Federation
1959-69	Honorary Secretary/Regional Chairman of the Far East and Australian Region
1977	Named Patron of the International Planned Parenthood Federation

References

1. UN Demographic Yearbook (1961).
2. Population Reference Bureau, *1991 World Population Data Sheet* (Washington, DC, 1991).
3. *The Straits Times*, "Survey on why some don't want three or more" (25 November 1989).

Chapter 6
Zahia Marzouk (1906 – 1988)

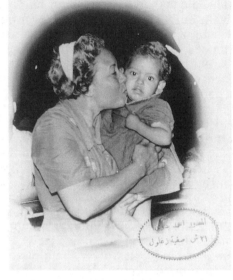

*Zahia Marzouk, founder of the Alexandria Family Planning
Association and the Happy Childhood Association, circa 1950.*

She would not allow women to do less than they were capable of

When Egypt regained its independence following the British
Protectorate in 1922, its population was estimated at 13.5 million people. Subsequent investments in public health and sani-
tation substantially decreased infant mortality and increased
longevity, resulting in an annual population growth rate of 2.9
per cent. Egypt's current population is 55 million. That figure
may reach 105 million by 2025.[1] Demographic trends are a
crucial factor in Egyptian social and economic policies. Ninety
per cent of Egypt's land comprises sand dunes and stony,
sandy plains. It is the narrow Nile Valley which sustains all life.
From its origins deep in Africa, the Nile River winds its way

northward to the Mediterranean nourishing people, livestock, farmlands and wildlife. But the fertile river valley and its delta are a mere 3.5 per cent of Egypt's land surface, and urban or village sprawl diminishes it year after year. Land reclamation and irrigation schemes abound, but more land is needed for new homes and village expansion. Indeed, there is little hope that Egypt's agricultural land will be able to provide for its growing population. The same is true for the labour market, which has not kept pace with burgeoning population. Egypt is dependent on emmigrant labour to lessen unemployment pressures and to send remittances to families left at home. Before the Gulf crisis of 1990, an estimated 3.5 million Egyptians worked abroad. Their wages represented a significant contribution to the national economy.

When Zahia Marzouk founded the first family planning association in Egypt, in the Mediterranean port of Alexandria, in 1962, she was well aware of the demographic trends of her country. Her main concern, however, was for women's health and well-being – in her view essential if the quality of life of Egypt's families was to improve. Her life-long commitment to this goal led her to create several institutions for service to family welfare: the Happy Childhood Association, the Institute for Training and Research in Family Planning, the Alexandria Family Planning Association and the Regional Federation of Social Services.

Zahia Marzouk was a social worker, administrator, painter, sculptress and mentor to many. I first met her in 1975 at the home of a friend. She was visiting Washington with a delegation of women who had attended the International Women's Year Conference in Mexico City. As she left she turned and said, "If you ever come to Egypt, just take a train to Alexandria; when you get off, ask any child to take you to Zahia Marzouk's home." A year later, I travelled to Egypt on an assignment and did indeed visit Mrs Marzouk. Our meeting took place on the terrace of the Palestine Hotel in Alexandria the first day of June. Mrs Marzouk was about to celebrate her 70th birthday and joked about how young she felt. A woman of remarkable vitality, dressed in trousers and a bright blouse, she had taken me on a tour of Alexandria's central market. There, she bantered with shop-keepers, teased the young salesmen and charmed all those we encountered.

She enjoyed talking about her life, her work and most recent projects. I feel fortunate to have had the opportunity to meet her, for she passed away in 1988.

In the autumn of 1990 I travelled to Alexandria once again to meet her colleagues, friends and family. Fifteen years separate her words and those of her admirers in this chapter.

Zahia Marzouk

"My father died when I was three years old. Mother was very courageous and although she herself was illiterate, she managed to educate my two sisters and me. My sisters wanted to get married. Not me; I wanted to study more. But that was virtually impossible for girls at the time. There was much discussion over whether or not girls should be educated. And the veil, how I resented wearing it. I put it on at 14 but often stood in front of the family and refused to wear it. One solution was to travel to school in a car so no one could see me. I stopped wearing the veil when I was sixteen [in the same year, 1923, that Huda Sharaawi publicly discarded her veil at Cairo Railway Station on her return from the International Feminist Conference at Rome]. Of course I was the terror of the family, always the cause of long discussions and problems but I insisted that I wouldn't wear it. I'd cover my hair, never mind that, but I'd never put a veil on my face!

"When I completed my schooling at the Teacher Training Institute, the family wanted me to stay at home, saying I didn't need money so why should I work. I wanted to continue my studies, to go away, to see the world. But I had to wait. In those days the university was not yet open to girls. Shortly after my graduation that changed, but it was too late for me.

"I wanted to teach. Nobody in the family understood why. They said, 'Why should you want to work if you don't need the money?' I insisted; I had a very strong will then. It was my uncle, my father's brother, who encouraged me – not openly – subtly. He didn't say much but he did not object to my ideas. That helped me a great deal.

"First I was appointed a teacher by the Ministry of Education. When they realized I was a good teacher, they chose me for further study – at the Royal Normal College in London! Once again my uncle helped out. He had studied in England so he planned everything. My mother didn't know a thing about my plans until the day I left. I travelled to Port Said to take a ship; it was the first time I had ever travelled alone. I didn't know what to do. I was afraid of everybody. I got through customs formalities, sailed to England, assured that I would be met by someone from the Education Office. To my surprise the person turned out to be the former headmistress of the training college from which I had graduated. She was very kind. I lodged in a hostel which was run by a woman professor. She gave me invaluable advice about English traditions and behaviour. There were so many strange customs to learn.

"When I returned to Egypt in 1931 I was appointed to a teachers' college. I taught psychology to a class of advanced teacher training students. And in 1933 I was selected to study abroad again. I became the first Egyptian woman to study in the United States. I attended the Harvard Graduate School of Education and studied psychology, problem children and medical social work. When I finished the courses I did field work in the mountains of Kentucky and Missouri where I worked with native Americans and the rural poor. It was a wonderful experience because when I returned to Egypt in 1935, I realized how little social work was being done here. I opened the first School of Social Work in Alexandria and in Cairo in 1936. By the next year we formed an association for social studies and in 1938 the Ministry of Social Affairs was created. When I first returned, I worked as a psychiatric social worker at the Ministry of Education. It created a stir; many objected. There were no women in Ministries at the time. But I succeeded in convincing them to let me stay.

"In 1937 we began to think about the population explosion. University professors, gynaecologists, statisticians, geologists, all sorts of people were interested in the future population of Egypt. We formed a small, unofficial association to discuss demographic issues. We wanted to hold a conference but thought it best to consult a religious person. Fortunately, the religious authority we contacted did not disapprove of family planning. He believed it was necessary if the woman's or child's life was in danger or if they were afraid of being in a very poor, needy situation. Based on his opinion, we went ahead and held a conference on population issues in 1937. It was sponsored by the Medical Association.

"Excellent papers were presented on a diversity of subjects. But no woman dared to give a presentation on the woman's view of family planning. You can imagine how controversial it was. The religious leaders disapproved, saying it was disgraceful for a woman to stand in public and talk about family planning. Everybody advised me not to do it, but it had to be done. My lecture was very successful. I approached the subject from the human side, saying that family planning provides protection for everyone and contributes to the child's well-being. Planned parenthood gives children what they need and it protects family life. When I began, they threw tomatoes at me, even eggs; but when I finished, I had convinced them. There was a good deal of applause.

"From the Ministry of Education I was transferred to the Ministry of Social Affairs where I was named Director of the Department of Social Agencies. All private agencies in Egypt were under my supervision. I also taught at the School of Social Work. In fact, most of the people working in the social welfare field now were once my students, even the under-secretaries. From my vantage point in the Ministry of Social Affairs I identified problems and then tried to find a way to address them. I initiated the formation of the Federation for Child Welfare and then created the Federation for Family Welfare.

"When I was named to the Ministry office in Alexandria I had even more opportunity to undertake new ideas. I was concerned about working mothers so I created day-care centres and, subsequently, night-care centres for mothers who, like nurses, work on night shifts. I went to Germany and negotiated a contract with the International Federation for Disabled and Physiotherapy to get assistance and approval to create a school for physiotherapy here. It was the first in Egypt. I also founded an institution for disabled children who need physiotherapy. Then I thought of the elderly because in 1936–38, average longevity was 37 years. Forty years later, because of health care and medical progress, people are living longer. We have many elderly people who have no one to care for them. I founded the first institution for old men, especially for those whose wives had died.

"I began to witness problems that mentally retarded children create for a normal family, so I created an institution for retarded children. We worked on tuberculosis and all infectious diseases. I was the first to call for a training and vocational institution for leprosy patients. We raised the money from private sources, from individuals. We collected from the wealthy, and sometimes the government contributed. But in the beginning it was always a voluntary effort. I became a fund-raiser.

"Now we are working on a new project. I formed a co-operative society to help older women. We have set up a co-operative day-care centre where the older women can feel useful when they help with the children. We are going to open a school to teach girls to be kindergarten minders and saleswomen. You see, there is a new generation with new needs. They are not living in the same conditions we knew as girls. It is a different society, with different attitudes and behaviour. We must try to understand the changes and help the younger generation.

"The problem in Egypt is that men still don't understand that women can do something valid. They think that once a woman gets married she's of no use. That she shouldn't work. They think that once a woman is married she must sit down, cook and take care of her children, her husband. But why should you educate a girl to go to university and then keep her inside the house? It is ridiculous. You are putting ability in prison. Men must change. I made a survey of working mothers and found that very few men help their wives. Of 750 working mothers, I found only 1.3 per cent of men were helping their wives, even though they benefit from her salary. And women must believe in themselves. They must be educated to know and *use* their rights. I don't believe religious people have anything to do with women's emancipation. Once a woman is convinced that she has rights, no religious person can stop her from having them.

In the family planning programme we are trying to teach the value of women *to women themselves* and to young people. We ask the children 'Why should a mother have so many children, why she should have a quarter of a loaf of bread instead of half a loaf?' We relate family planning to the responsiblities of family life, to having sufficient resources for supporting a family. We've started training courses on family life education for teachers. We teach them that contraception goes back to ancient Egyptian times. Honey, the rock of the crocodile and the dachka, a condom made out of thin skin, were all used then. We want to educate people on modern contraception, better ways than those passed on from grandmothers. We find that women talk openly with other women about sexual things but not with their husbands. This is one of the problems we have to deal with. Marriage should be an understanding between a man and a woman. Living together, satisfying each other, is part of the agreement. But it is difficult to get husband and wife to talk about sexuality or about family planning.

"I got married in 1934 when I first came back to Egypt from the US. We met at Harvard. I didn't know him before and I never thought of getting married to him. When we came back to Egypt he went one way and I another. We didn't see each other for some time. When we did meet again we realized we had something in common. We married and built our own house. My husband is a nice man. He always encouraged me. He still does, otherwise I wouldn't be here, leaving him all alone in the house while I talk with you.

"One reason I was able to do the things I've mentioned is because people warm to me easily, they like me. It is part of my character. People write when they are in trouble; they phone and say, 'We are in trouble, what can we do?' They come up to me in the street or in shops. I was like this from the time I was born. Even when I was a young girl at school, I had to do things for other people. I would see somebody crying and I would go and find out why. I was born with a humanitarian side in me. If I look back on my life, I have the great satisfaction of never doing anything that I did not like. All my life was a continuous pleasure – satisfying people, loving them and having them love me in return. I am a happy woman, don't I look it?"

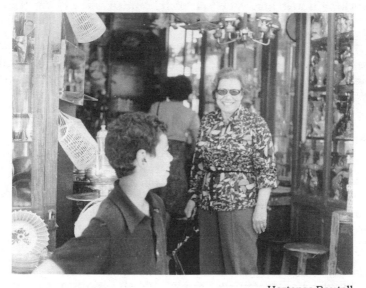

Hortense Boutell

Zahia Marzouk visiting the markets of Alexandria in 1976.

Dr Salha Awad

The grounds of the Institute for Training and Research in Family Planning seemed like a quiet oasis amidst the hustle of Alexandria's teeming side streets in the autumn of 1990. Dr Salha Awad, president of the Institute, was seated at her desk behind which a photograph of Zahia Marzouk smiled from the wall above. Dr Awad is also the president of the Alexandria Family Planning Association which Zahia Marzouk founded. It was as a young employee of the Ministry of Social Affairs in Alexandria that she met Zahia Marzouk.

"Mrs. Marzouk had the courage to do things that others wouldn't dare take on. If she believed in something she would keep at it until she succeeded. That is why she was a pioneer in so many things. She never hesitated to do something because it might be unpopular with superiors or jeopardize her job, or put her in a difficult situation. She would never be stopped by routine or procedures. She was very creative and possessed a good imagination, always willing to try something new, take a risk. For a government employee, that was unusual.

"Of course this made her controversial. Many men resented working under her. When she was named Director for Voluntary Associations in the Ministry of Social Affairs, the biggest department in the Ministry, some men resigned or asked to be transferred to other agencies. In a way she benefitted from being a pioneer. I think it was easier when there were so few women. But it was her personality and her character which were the driving forces behind her achievements. Intelligent and broad-minded, she had the courage to express herself no matter what. She would go to the very end to take her ideas to others and convince them.

"One of her favourite stories was about how she managed to work towards the abolition of prostitution, which had been legal in Egypt until the 1930s. One of her tasks in the Ministry of Social Affairs was to recommend what should be done about houses of prostitution. Since she knew nothing about it herself she decided to live in the prostitutes' district in Cairo for a week. She wanted to observe how the 'business' worked, to understand the system. At first she was afraid they would discover that she was an official from the Ministry. Eventually she had to tell the 'boss' that she was there to study the situation. She gathered the information she needed and spearheaded the abolition of legal prostitution in Egypt. This is another pioneering idea she had. And I believe this was before she was married. Her husband didn't mind what others said because she fascinated him, so much energy, so many ideas, such creativity.

"As a creative person she had lots of ideas but she needed other skills to implement them. The practical realization of ideas was not one of her strengths. But she was good at identifying people who could put her ideas into practice. If you understood her and knew how to work with her, it was very productive. When we started this Institute, neither of us knew how to set up such a training centre. People live here; it is almost like a hotel service. Neither of us had experience in this. We were experimenting, learning, trying to do this or that and if it didn't work we'd start again. She was always ready to try something and would never say, 'Oh no, it doesn't work', but try again from another angle.

"She created associations for all sorts of needs she identified. Many became part of the government's public policy. For example, she realized that the 'traditional' midwives needed training. But they were operating illegally and were in hiding from officials. She sent researchers to find out who and where they were. She then designed a training course and convinced them to attend. Eventually she persuaded the government to license them and the training programme was adopted by the Ministry of Health. Another example was Zahia's dislike of the word orphanage. She felt it was demeaning to children. In our society, it is a disgrace, a catastrophe to have a child out of marriage. Abandoned children are found in trash cans, on the doorsteps of mosques or churches. The young mothers leave their families, abandon the newborn and try to find work somewhere. Zahia used her influence to get the abandoned children turned over to a private orphanage called the Happy Childhood Association. The idea was to provide a school for the children from a very early age and right on up to higher education, or training or marriage.

"At the Family Planning Association we have a programme called Rural Women Pioneers. We select village women who can read and write, are interested in community problems and want to help as volunteers. They educate their communities in health care, nutrition, hygiene, childcare, and family planning. It is a very successful programme. This is another legacy of Zahia Marzouk. She would not allow women to do less than they were capable of.

"It seems that Zahia had heard that her father wanted his second child to be a boy. In fact he fathered three daughters. Maybe her motivation consisted of showing her father that even though she was female, she could do just as well as any son? I don't know, but it is possible."

Laila Souka

Laila Souka is the Director of the Happy Childhood Association. It functions as a day care centre for working mothers, a home for orphaned children, a training centre for social workers, a kindergarten and a toy-making co-operative. Hired by Zahia Marzouk when she finished her social work training, Mrs Souka now directs a staff of 80.

"I had heard about Mrs Marzouk when I was a student. She was known as a strong and clever woman. When I finished my studies, the Director of the Institute for Social Work sent me here to apply for a job. I was frightened at the idea of meeting her but she greeted me with a smile and my fear vanished. At the time I hadn't thought beyond just getting a job for awhile. After working with Mrs Marzouk I changed my mind. I saw that I could be much more, achieve much more. 'Always think about others', she said, 'not about yourself. You will be happy when others are happy.'"She made you feel as though you were a leader in your work. She made you feel responsible.

"Working with her was a wonderful experience – so much so that now I find it very difficult to work with others. She knew people well. She could see inside you and know what you were thinking. If she believed you were clever, she pushed you. She encouraged me to get a Masters Degree and gave me the chance to study in Cairo, in 1974. She would help anyone – all her employees – with their personal life. She allowed employees to bring their children to the nursery here, free. It was very far-sighted, a day-care provision for employees. Once when the government raised salaries by 20 per cent for all civil service employees, Mrs Marzouk wouldn't let us be left out. She gave us a 20 per cent raise out of her own pocket, until she could convince the government that private agencies should have the salary raises as well.

"She loved children and wanted all children to have a family. She convinced the police department to bring us the abandoned children who are turned over to the police. We keep them here until we find a suitable foster family. We have placed over two thousand children. Right now we have 30 babies waiting to be placed.

"Her biggest influence on me was to teach me to work hard, to have a sense of responsibility. From her I learned to be self confident, not to depend on men. She taught us that women can handle anything. Mrs Marzouk is living in all of us. She is still here in all the people whom she taught."

Dr Hafes Youssuf

Dr Youssuf is the director of another of Zahia Marzouk's creations: the Model Comprehensive Clinic for Family Planning. It is there we met and talked about Mrs Marzouk's legacy. A well-known gynaecologist, Dr Youssuf has written extensively on sexuality and sex education in Egypt.

"I first met Mrs Marzouk in 1962 when she was Under-Secretary at the Ministry of Social Affairs. Before that, as an ordinary person in Alexandria, I had heard about a woman who was very active in social causes. Then a friend contacted me, saying that Mrs Marzouk was going to open a family planning clinic in a neighborhood of Alexandria. He asked if I would be interested in working in a family planning centre. I was then 28 years old and had been working as a gynaecologist for several years. I accepted and he took me to meet Mrs Marzouk. It was a peculiar visit. She asked me very few questions and said, 'Okay, go and get started.'

"But the clinic had to be set up, started from scratch. After about two weeks she asked me how I was doing. But she knew; she had seen what I had started and was pleased. She never said so, but I could see it in her face. She never suppressed her students or those with whom she worked. She encouraged us to try new things, new ideas.

"She has left a group of independent thinkers and doers as her legacy. All of us, Dr Awad, Mrs Souka, myself and many more. She created independent people; she didn't want to keep us under her wing or control us. She wanted us to go out and do.

"Active people like her arouse the jealousy of others, particularly men. Because she was pushing herself into the male field, was very active and effective, those who couldn't keep up would speak against her out of jealousy. She was the most courageous woman I have known, and she was certainly more courageous than many men I know. This courage was what attracted me and convinced me to stay on and work in family planning. In 1970 I was qualified to teach at the University but I decided to work with her instead."

Kamel Marzouk

The teenage Zahia who greeted me at the Marzouk family home seems to have inherited the energy and sparkling eyes of her grandmother. She guided me from room to room pointing out her grandmother's memorabilia: awards, photographs, paintings or sculptures carved and polished by the elder Zahia. We then sat with her grandfather, Kamel Marzouk, a giant of an octogenarian, who was pleased at the opportunity of talking about his beloved wife.

"We met in Boston where we were both students. At one point

her scholarship cheque had not arrived. She hadn't eaten for two days. Through the window of a cafeteria she saw a couple of young Egyptians, a friend and me. She came in, introduced herself and told us of her plight. Of course we offered to pay for her meal. She thanked us, ordered a huge dinner, ate in silence and then got up and said goodbye. We were amazed by this audacious behaviour from an Egyptian girl.

"It had been arranged that I marry a cousin. When I told my family that I wanted to marry Zahia, they laughed at me and at the fact that I would marry a working woman. They teased me for a long time.

"We had a wonderful life together. The social life of Alexandria revolved around us, we gave great parties and often the great singer, Umm Kolthoum, came. She and Zahia were close friends. Everyone came to our house, kings, prime ministers; she knew everybody.

"She led a life of service to others. We still encounter people who tell us that she helped them out financially and we don't understand how she did it because we never knew and she was not a rich person at all.

"She didn't care what other people thought or what they said; she was so sure of herself and her goals that the rest didn't matter. Somehow she wanted to prove that she could do as much as anyone else, if not more. She was so busy helping people that finally her heart overtired. She couldn't keep going. There is such an empty place in my life now – no one can ever fill it or make it less painful."

Zahia Ahmad Metwaly Marzouk

1906   Born Alexandria, Egypt
1929   Received Teachers Diploma, Egypt
1931   Royal Normal College, London, teaching diploma
1934   Harvard School of Education, diploma in education of special handicapped groups
1935–36 Opened first School of Social Work in Alexandria and then Cairo
1962   Creates the Alexandria Family Planning Association
1963–66 Under-Secretary for Social Affairs, Alexandria. Creates numerous welfare organizations
1947–78 Received dozens of awards in recognition of contributions to social work, child welfare and family planning

References

1. Population Reference Bureau, *1991 World Population Data Sheet* (Washington, DC, 1991).

Chapter 7
Dr M.L. Kashetra Snidvongs
(b. 1908)

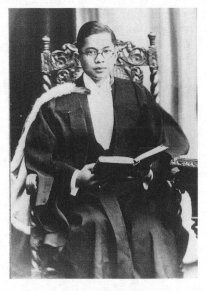

M.L. Kashetra Snidvongs as a student at the University of Durham, England, in 1930.

Honest mentor to an entire generation

When the young Dr M.L. Kashetra Snidvongs returned to his native Siam in the mid 1930s, following studies at Durham University, the kingdom's population stood at 8.1 million people. Siam became Thailand in 1939, after the *coup d'état* of 1935 ended the absolute monarchy. Today Thais number 58.8 million.[1] This formidable increase in human numbers, due in part to improvements in public health services following the end of World War II, took place despite the remarkable efforts of non-governmental and governmental agencies in reducing the population growth rate from 3.3 to 1.3 per cent.

The story of family planning in Thailand is complex. As early as 1955 medical personnel and concerned social activists began providing family planning guidance and services in a small clinic in the old city of Bangkok. This led to the registration of the Family Planning Association of Thailand in August 1958. Yet government policy lagged far behind these first visionaries. The following chapter is a tribute to a founder of another non-governmental family planning organization, the Planned Parenthood Federation of Thailand. Known to all, affectionately, as Dr Kaset, the octogenarian professor is most admired for his efforts to provide the best possible education to those Thai medical students who are leaders of the medical community today.

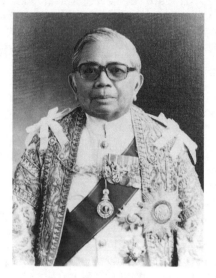

M.L. Kashetra Snidvongs, mentor to a generation of medical doctors, in Thailand, 1990.

As a Professor of Medicine and a University Dean, he spent most of his career assigned to the Red Cross Hospital in the grounds of Chulalongkorn University. Still Chairman of the Red Cross Children's Fund, which is an orphanage for abandoned children, Dr Kaset is very proud of his forty-year service with the Red Cross. Indeed, the International Red Cross has given him their highest award, the Henry Dunant Medal. Unfortunately Dr Kaset was in poor health when I visited Bangkok in the spring of 1991, but he remains both controversial and influential in Thai society. Even in his old age he is a fighting man.

The accomplishments of family planners in reducing the population growth rate of Thailand are soon to be dwarfed by the effort needed to confront a growing crisis in Thailand, that of the spread of HIV. Currently there are an estimated 300,000 individuals who are HIV positive. Based on infection projections, this figure will jump to 6 million before the end of the decade.[2] According to the Bangkok newspaper *Nation*, a survey on the spread of AIDS in Thailand indicates that the disease is spreading faster in the rural north than in Bangkok and other areas. The survey revealed that in rural districts, 50 per cent of people had their first sexual experience before 16 and 73 per cent gained this experience with a prostitute. The case for safe sex education cannot be made more eloquently.

Professor Charas Suwanwela

Professor Charas is the respected President of Chulalongkorn University, a neurosurgeon, and administrator. Our conversation took place in the elegant sitting-room of his offices at the university. A tall man with a confident stride, Professor Charas told me he manages to treat patients despite his administrative duties. He expressed gratitude for the opportunity to speak about his mentor.

"Dr. Kaset was my teacher but far more than just that to me. He was instrumental in my whole career. He has many connections, family connections and one of those is with Her Majesty. He is the older brother of Her Majesty's mother. Although they had different mothers, he is considered to be an uncle to the Queen. He was the Royal Family's obstetrician and advisor to the King on health matters.

"When I graduated from medical school in 1955, he asked the King to establish a scholarship for leading medical graduates to study abroad, to improve their medical knowledge. The idea was similar to that of His Majesty's father who established higher education in this country. His father created Chulalongkorn University and gave scholarships to young Thais to go abroad and return to this university. These scholarships disappeared when the father died. When His Majesty revived them I was the first to be given that opportunity. Dr Kaset petitioned the King to give me the scholarship.

"Abroad I studied my selected area, surgery. I was trained in neurosurgery and came back to Thailand in 1961. When I returned Dr Kaset became Dean of the Medical School and director of the hospital. Before that he had been Head of the Department of Obstetrics and Gynaecology at Chulalongkorn Hospital. Dr Kaset made a significant contribution in developing the field of gynaecology in this country by sending people abroad for training. When I came back to Chulalongkorn Hospital, it already had a very big family planning unit. People from all over the country were coming here for IUD insertion. He had taken over a ward which was no longer used and turned it into a family planning service. I remember that at the time, the Prime Minister and the Deputy Prime Minister were saying that Thailand needed a lot more people if Thailand was to become a strong country. So what Dr Kaset was doing was definitely against the government's policy but it went on because of the support of the public.

"Fortunately for Thailand, we are a tolerant people, we accept things very easily. There is nothing in the religion which is against family planning. Abortion is not accepted because one of the five major sins in Buddhism is killing, so abortion is considered to be something very unacceptable. Abortion is illegal here. We accept abortion only on medical grounds. There was an attempt to pass a law to permit abortion on social grounds but it did not pass. But no one had made the decision about IUDs, whether or not they are abortive; that is the technical side.

"Dr Kaset recognized the need for family planning and he had the courage to carry through by providing services. It was very important at the time because it was several more years before the official policy was changed and services made available on a large scale. Since he was well respected, partly because of being the Dean and then the Director of the second largest hospital in Thailand, and because of his connections with the Royal Family, he was able to have a lot of influence on the society. If someone else had started the family planning programme at that point, it might not have got through. Later he was appointed to the Parliament and made his ideas well known. Although not directly involved, I think he was very influential in turning national policy around, in setting policy.

"Dr Kaset is a mixture of many things. He stands out as a man of principle. He went through many stages in his life and always stood by his principles. He influenced many of us. The second man who received a scholarship was Dr Prawase; both of us remain very close to Dr Kaset. Dr Prawase is the most respected social advocate in the country. He dares to say to the government, 'This is wrong.' He was appointed by the last government to be an advisor; he turned it down because he doesn't agree with the government in many areas. We both feel very close to Dr Kaset because we are the earlier ones to benefit from his guidance. When we were studying abroad he was the one who really looked after our well-being. After we came back he nurtured us, helping us to develop in our own area.

"I owe a lot to him. For example, when I left to study neurosurgery, no one knew what neurosurgery was. But by the time I returned from my studies in 1961, there was a new facility at the Hospital to house neurology, neurosurgery and psychiatry. Dr Kaset had asked the Bangkok Bank to build an entire new unit for treating neurological disorders. As soon as I came back I had all these facilities for my work. That just shows how much he looked after us."

Professor Nikorn Dusitin

Dr Nikorn, who is Head of the Department of Obstetrics and Gynaecology at Chulalongkorn University, asked if we could meet at his office at the University Medical Faculty. It was early morning, prior to his rounds in the wards of the hospital. He reminisced about the early days of the family planning with more than a touch of humour.

"Dr Kaset was a great teacher. The first thing I remember about him was his courage to go against what was accepted at the time. He was the Head of the Department when I was a young staff member, about 1960. At the time, interns and residents performed tubal ligations after three, and sometimes two, pregnancies if there was a good cause to do so. The two other big hospitals, including the largest maternity hospital in the country, refused to do tubal ligation before four children, but here at Chulalongkorn, Dr Kaset believed that the poor, if they had good reason, could choose. So women would go to the Women's Hospital for the first two children and then, for the third, come here to Chulalongkorn to have their tubal ligation. He was concerned about the situation of the poor and their ability to feed more children. That was his motivation. Three children were already too many for some families, why should they have more?

"In those days communications and transportation systems were not well developed. We received many patients from the eastern seaboard of the country. They had to come by boat, then hire a truck and often we would receive women in terrible condition following childbirth – with septicaemia, haemorrhaging, obstructed labour. People came from all over the country. Sometimes the people had been travelling for days, if not many long hours, to bring a desperate case to us, by boat, truck or whatever. In fact, as interns, when we saw a truck arriving we would gear up for the worst, knowing it would be a woman in desperate shape, oftentimes dead upon arrival. So you see, if we did a tubal ligation it was in a way the only method for saving a woman who should not have another pregnancy. We saw, for example, a lot of cases of hypertension. There were only three big hospitals in the city and everyone would refer their patients to us. We had so many requests for ligations that the operating room became known as the ligation room. We worked very hard.

"It wasn't long before I was given a scholarship to study in the US. For the last year, it was a Population Council fellowship. I think I was one of the first doctors from Thailand to receive this. When the Population Council invited Dr Kaset to visit America, for a meeting on IUDs at the Population Council, he called me up. Knowing that I would be returning home soon, he asked if I would work with him and Dr Aree in family planning. I agreed and when I returned in 1967 we opened a clinic which was described as a 'research clinic'. But we didn't do research; we placed IUDs. We had to be discreet about our work because many people believed the country needed a larger population, more soldiers to protect it. If we had operated openly there would have been lots of opposition. There were rumors that IUDs could cause cancer. And for decades now, there have been those who accuse doctors of using the Thai people as guinea pigs. They accuse us of believing that whatever the foreigners say is good and we just go ahead and use it.

"We wanted to do clinical research to prove once and for all that IUDs are safe. Indeed, after the clinic had been going for two or three years, I proposed that we establish a research centre in gynaecology and family planning. Dr Kaset helped me establish the centre and a few years later it was recognized by the World Health Organization as a collaborative research centre in human reproduction. It is a very important centre in the WHO reproductive health research network.

"The first day we officially opened the Research Clinic four or five ladies came. Dr Kaset arrived and saw the women waiting on the bench so he took one of them in the examination room and asked the nurse to prepare her, put her on the examining table. He did the examination; all was well so he inserted the IUD. He then began explaining about the IUD. She replied, 'But doctor, I came here for something else.' All the others had come for an IUD but not her. You see, in Thailand, people respect doctors so much – at least in those days – that she hadn't dared say anything at first. He asked if she wanted the IUD removed and she said, 'No, it's all right, I'll keep it.' That is the story of the first IUD placed by our clinic. Soon enough news of our clinic – 'where you could get IUDs' – got around through word of mouth and we had so many patients we couldn't keep up with the demand.

"We had received about 300 IUDs and had expected that the supply would last about six months. Within a few weeks, we had run out and had to request more. People came from all over the country. Word of mouth only. We then received three or four thousand IUDs but even they didn't last very long. People would come at four or five in the morning, waiting in front of the clinic until one or two o'clock, when the clinic opened. We heard that it was the largest IUD clinic in the world with two hundred IUDs inserted every afternoon. We worked like an assembly line with three tables. The nurse would be waiting beside the client, the doctor would come and do the examination to see if all was right and then insert the IUD. In those days we were just three doctors running the clinic, we called ourselves the three musketeers. Dr Aree was the leader, then a classmate of mine and me.

"As you know, Thais are very entrepreneurial. We discovered that someone had begun to organize a tour to Bangkok for 50 Bahts. You could come from a province in the northeast, arrive in Bangkok early in the morning, go to visit the Palace and in the afternoon you visited the clinic for an IUD insertion. All for 50 bahts. We didn't know a thing about it until one day one of the women who had come was pregnant so we refused to insert the IUD. We said, 'We are sorry but you must come back again when you have had your child.' She looked up and said, 'Can I get a refund, then?' What refund? It was a free clinic; there was no charge for our services. That is how we discovered that for 50 bahts you could tour Bangkok and have an IUD as well.

"We had hoped to keep good records, to do research on the IUDs and all, but we were too busy, we had to abandon any hope of research just to keep up with the daily demand for insertions. In those days, not many people thought this was a good idea. Especially the deputy Director of the hospital, a woman trained in the Philippines. She didn't like the IUD idea at all. She didn't think it was needed. She was from a very high status family and she didn't like the fact that so many people came and lined up body to body, waiting their turn. She said, 'This disgusts me that women line up like this; it is disgraceful.' But we didn't know how to do otherwise because all we had was a small room. If it hadn't been for Dr Kaset, we would have been turned out of that hospital ward. Also, because of the unexpected success of this service we needed more funds from the hospital's budget.

"The number of requests for tubal ligations increased rapidly because word got around that we were willing to do them. We tried to get the husband's consent for tubal ligations but if not, it was permissible if the woman wanted it. It was not illegal. Women here have a lot of character and make many decisions in the home.

"Dr Kaset was always concerned about others' hardships. He traveled all around the provinces trying to keep aware of medical needs, the facilities there where people are very poor. He was concerned that people should be treated there where they lived, for they couldn't afford to come to the city hospitals. In later years he got a mobile unit and used to go around and talk with people in the villages himself, attempting to keep abreast of the needs.

"Dr Kaset looks very serious, even gruff, but he is a very kind-hearted man. When he would give students the oral examination he would threaten them jokingly with an ashtray if they didn't give the right answer – but that was his way of demanding excellence."

Dr Aree Somboonsuk

Dr Aree Somboonsuk has been President of Planned Parenthood Association of Thailand (PPAT) since 1985 and was one of its founders in 1969. Our conversation took place over lunch; he had invited me to join him at the Royal Thai Sporting Club where our table overlooked the race track.

"I think the thing that motivated Dr Kaset was the fact that when he was born, the Thai population was only about 10 million. He has seen everything – from 10 million – up to now. At the time when we opened family planning clinics the population was about 24 million. That was when the government began to act. Every morning when Dr Kaset made his rounds in the hospital he would ask the mothers 'How many children do you have?' Many would answer 'Ten or twelve'. One day he counted the number of children born to the women who were in the six beds of one hospital ward and it reached nearly one hundred. So every morning when he did his walk-around with the students he would tell them, 'You see, that is going to be our problem in the future.'

"He was concerned about women's health: in medical textbooks it is well-documented that after the fourth child you enter the high-risk group. Women need the time to recover from one pregnancy before another. He was concerned about all these things. In the old days there was virtually no abortion; it is against our religion and our traditional concepts. Nowadays in the obstetric and gynaecological wards, we see the results of quack abortions. Women come to us once they have been unsuccessfully treated by illegal means. Many of them are nearly dead due to septicaemia, infections and bleeding. Abortion existed before, of course, but it was not as frequent. This, too, influenced Dr Kaset.

"His commitment to others, to the poor, is interesting because he is a member of the royal family. He bears the title ML, which is a royal title. He was sent abroad on scholarship by King Rama VI who was the founder of Chulalongkorn Hospital. Dr Kaset wanted to pay back the advantages he received, give something back to the hospital and to the country as well. As soon as he returned from Britain, and until now, he has been caring for the hospital and its people. I first met him as his student and was later appointed a staff member in his department; I have been with him ever since.

"We started the family planning association in 1965 but we had been doing it for a long time before – tubectomies, IUDs and family planning methods – without having official organization. But when we felt the time had come for having an official association, we opened in 1965. Tubectomies had been permitted but not unless the woman had six children already. We did them after four. The government began to get interested in family planning and population policies when the World Bank analysed our economic situation. Their study pointed out that if the population growth rate was not dealt with, we would have unemployment problems in the future. That was in 1957. After that there were three national seminars held on the population question. The first one concluded, 'Let things be, nature will take care of it'. But the academic people said, 'No, we have to do more.' On 17 March 1970 the government set forth its population policy and less than one month later the Planned Parenthood Association of Thailand became a legal entity, on 14 April 1970. We had applied before, but since there was no government policy we had to wait.

"Dr Kaset was involved in the second and third national seminars and had much influence on the debates. Also, all the foreign visitors who came to Thailand to look at the population question, came to see him. He got money from the Population Council for research and from the IPPF for the mobile units. We would contact the governors, especially the wives of the governors and everything would be arranged by the time the mobile unit reached the village. All this was before the government programme became a reality, so we had to have friends in the provinces helping us.

"Once the government became involved it was apparent that it didn't have well trained or equipped staff for family planning. And many Thais were still reluctant; they hung on to the old ideas of a large population being necessary for the country. So we started a series of seminars for the high-ranking officers of the ministries, governors, deputy governors, politicians. The idea was to tell them what we were doing, to explain the benefits of family planning to individuals and to the country. This process took nearly five years – to reach all the governors and high officials throughout the entire kingdom. We believed that if they knew the facts they would be ready to help us. The most important was the wives. They all had to be members of the Red Cross, since the Governors were chief of the Red Cross in each province. Dr Kaset would call up the wives and tell them about family planning, what the problems were for other women. Since they knew the difficulties of having four or five children themselves, they were very interested in learning about family planning and thus in supporting our efforts for others as well. We knew that when we got the wife of the Governor to help, we would have the co-operation of the Governor assured.

"We also did a lot of training of grassroots volunteers. The Red Cross had some 20 health stations throughout the country whereas the government had only a few. This was our duty,

to help people, but we didn't have enough supplies to help
everyone; that was the government's duty. Later on when
government became active, we helped in service delivery in
remote areas, there where it had no services. But the important
point in the old days was to change false reasoning about family
planning and population issues."

Professor Dr Prawase Wasi

Dr Prawase is a geneticist and Director of the Thalassaemia
Centre, at the Faculty of Medicine at Mahidol University. We
managed to arrange a meeting in the lobby of the Asia Hotel in
central Bangkok where he was to speak at a medical seminar.
Well-known and respected in Thailand for his uncompromising
honesty, Dr Prawase, in fact, mirrors the integrity of his early
mentor, Dr Kaset.

"I first met Dr Kaset in 1957. He was at the Medical School
but was also secretary of the King's Scholarship Fund. I was
a candidate for a scholarship and he was to interview me. Dr
Kaset recommended me to the King and it resulted in a grant
from the King's private fund to study in the United States.
From there I went to London to study genetics at University
College. He disciplined me even there because he used to go
around visiting King's scholars. When I returned to Thailand I
found he had already negotiated support for my research with
the China Medical Board, a part of the Rockefeller Foundation.
He had planned this even before I returned so that I would
have the support needed for my work. We became very close,
working together even though there is over 20 years between
us in age.
  "I came to know him intimately. We talked a lot about the
public interest, public welfare, politics and I found that he
abhors corruption and abuse of public confidence. He cannot
tolerate corruption and he urged me to write about it. He is
very critical of corrupt officials, even his own relatives or people
in the palace. He is very straightforward in his opinions. He
was Secretary General of the Red Cross for many years and
he always demonstrated his concern for the poor. About 15
years ago, Chulalongkorn Hospital, which is the Red Cross
Hospital, was erecting a new building. Many people involved
wanted to have a lot of private rooms built. But Dr Kaset, as the
secretary said, 'No, only a few. We need rooms for the poor.' He
had to fight for this. The quarrel even became a national issue.

He does not hesitate to quarrel for what he believes in. And very often the matter gets to the King or the Queen because of this fighting.

"Very recently again, the new Secretary General of the Red Cross was appointed by the military as the Minister of University Affairs. Dr Kaset protested at a meeting in front of the Princess, very strongly. He had read in the Red Cross Charter that the Administrator of the Red Cross should not be involved in politics. So he insisted that the Secretary General had to resign. In Thailand there is a system of denouncing people by leaflet. When people don't like each other, they don't like to criticize publicly; they send out anonymous leaflets. Right after that meeting with the Princess, the very same day, there were leaflets denouncing Dr Kaset, saying how rude he had been in front of the Princess, how he had shouted at the Secretary General. I think this describes his personality.

"Whenever he is angry with somebody, he calls me and I go to see him, to let him express his anger.

"He is very much against corruption and wants to support good people. His anti-corruption attitude is not well-known to the public, but I know about it because we have been very close. Dr Charas, the rector of Chulalongkorn University, was the first king's scholar and Dr Kaset has supported him continuously because he is a good man. He was the one who recommended that the King establish the Anandamahidol Foundation. He was secretary of the medical division of the Foundation for a long time, until a very old age.

"In 1955 he recommended that the King create this scholarship and then a foundation in the name of his brother who had died in a accident at a very young age. The King had fond memories of his brother, so he created the foundation to send young Thais abroad to study. It gave scholarships for many disciplines, starting with medicine and science, the arts, agriculture, law. Each year they select top students for study abroad. There are over one hundred scholars in various fields. Dr Charas is one, myself, another. This was one of Dr Kaset's greatest contributions to Thai society, I believe, to provide the opportunity like this and then to provide the support when we returned to Thailand.

"Dr Kaset's concern with family planning is also a great contribution. It is well known that Thailand has been fairly successful in this area, from 3.3 per cent down to 1.5 per cent growth rate. Many people contributed to this success and Dr Kaset, himself, contributed greatly. At the beginning he was controversial; there were those opposed to family planning. They said, 'Oh, they want to prevent us from having many people in the country.' But resistance melted quickly. As a member of a noble family Dr Kaset was able to convince the King and the Queen that this was a concern that had to be addressed. He is straightforward, a dedicated but controversial person in Thai society."

Professor Dr M.L. Kashetra Snidvongs

1908	Born Bangkok, Thailand
1930	University of Durham, England MB, BS
1937	Staff doctor and Relief Officer, the Thai Red Cross Society, Chulalongkorn Hospital
1950–53	Served in Thai Armed Forces, South Korea
1955	Professor, Department of OBGYN, Faculty of Medicine, Chulalongkorn Hospital
1960	Dean of the Faculty of Medicine and Director of Chulalongkorn Hospital
1969	Council Member, Thai Red Cross Society
1989	Awarded Henry Dunant Medal from The Red Cross and Red Crescent, Geneva

References

1. Population Reference Bureau, *1991 World Population Data Sheet*, Washington, DC 1991
2. *South* magazine June/July 1991, and *International Herald Tribune*, 26 March 1991
3. *Le Monde*, 30 April 1991

Chapter 8
Dr Tewhida Ben Sheikh (b. 1909)

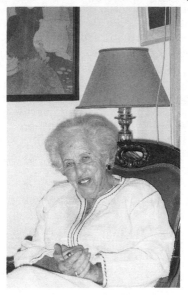

Dr Tewhida Ben Sheikh at home during the author's visit in 1990.

She listened to society; she listened to its people

Tunisia became a French colony in the late 19th century. The French colonial rule lasted a mere 70 years, but had great influence on the educated classes of modern Tunisia. A largely agricultural economy was managed by a colonial administration which controlled every sector of Tunisian society, except its cultural and religious life. Indeed, maintaining strong traditions was one way the colonized people maintained their identity and dignity. Any breaks with tradition were, thus, considered both socially and politically unacceptable. In Tewhida Ben Sheikh's youth, Tunisian women were veiled on the rare occasions they left the protection of their homes. Few girls attended school and no girl completed secondary school. Marriages were arranged for the benefit of family ties and relationships; the bride's or groom's opinion held little weight in the choice of spouse.

Tewhida Ben Sheikh's young, widowed mother was remarkably courageous and far-sighted. She believed enough in her daughter's craving for education and public service that she was willing to break with tradition and "proper behaviour" to allow her daughter opportunities of which few even dreamed. Tewhida Ben Sheikh studied medicine at the Faculté de Medecine in Paris. She became a medical doctor in 1936. It would be another 10 years before a second Tunisian woman followed her to medical school.

Now retired, Dr Ben Sheikh lives in her family home on a tree-lined avenue in Tunis. We had arranged to meet at the IPPF Regional Offices. The appointment was set for nine in the morning and I had wanted to arrive before Dr Ben Sheikh so as to be there to welcome her. As I approached the entrance to the building a car pulled up; a woman in the passenger seat was waving to me. As I was to learn later from her colleagues, this punctual informality was part and parcel of Dr Ben Sheikh's style and her attitude towards work – and life. Dressed in pullover, white collar, pearls, a skirt and brown loafers, the famous doctor appeared more like a well-dressed college student. A small woman, barely five feet tall, she had the gait of a giant and I soon discovered that she was always ready to laugh. The tape of our conversation is full of laughter, self-mockery and amusing asides. Dr Ben Sheikh no doubt suffers fools poorly. Her hands would flail at futility when one mentioned beaucracy or politics; her eyes would moisten when talking of social miseries. The direction of her allegiance is not in doubt. Soon after we had installed ourselves in an upstairs meeting room, a woman colleague, Dr Aicha Chakroun arrived with a Zairian doctor settled in Tunisia, Dr Christopher Luleka Anicet. Both had come to pay tribute to their teacher and mentor.

Dr Tewhida Ben Sheikh

"I come from a well-known Tunisian family. I never knew my father; we were four children, three girls and a boy. The son was born after my father's death. I was thus raised by my mother who was a most extraordinary woman. She was educated in Arabic and did not speak French. She was a devout Muslim and very open minded. Despite the fact that she was alone, widowed young, she managed to see to it that all of us had secondary school educations. My sisters and I were the first Tunisian girls to complete secondary school. That's the way she was, my mother, she wanted us to go as far as *we* wanted in school. I was the first girl to pass the baccalauréat degree in Tunisia, in 1928. But, of course then came the question, what was I going to do with it?

"It was about then that I met a Russian woman, the wife of a well-known French doctor, Dr Burnet. He was the Deputy Director of the Pasteur Institute here in Tunis. His wife was a wonderful woman; she knew one of my professors at secondary school, who was interested in what I would do next. I wanted to do social work, help others; I thought I could work in one of the institutes or charities or the Pasteur Institute. So this woman suggested that I talk with her husband. Dr Etienne Burnet was a literary man, a philosopher who had studied Greek and Latin. He was also a famous medical researcher. I still remember going to see him. It was a summer day, in June or July. They lived on a hill in the Belvedere neighbourhood of Tunis. I went alone. It was 1929. I remember it so well. As soon as I arrived he asked, 'Now my little one, what is it you would *like* to do?' 'I would like to do something, perhaps study medicine,' I replied, 'but there is no medical school here in Tunis – so perhaps Algiers?' He looked at me; he hesitated, then said, 'My little one. If you want to accomplish something, to study medicine, you must enter by the big door. You must go to Paris.' I almost laughed. 'You are dreaming, sir.' 'I can help you,' he said, 'I know many people in Paris and can arrange for you to go there.' So I went home and told my mother, sisters and brother. My brother had received his baccalauréat at the same time as I, but my mother hadn't yet thought about sending him off to pursue university studies. I watched my mother's reaction to my story. She didn't reject it outright so I began to think that perhaps there was hope.

"My mother had never left Tunisia, but she was very broad-minded and very courageous. Everyone – her mother, brothers, sisters – all of them said she shouldn't let me go. In the meantime Dr Burnet started writing to his friends in Paris to try to find a family in which I could live while I studied. Finally he found an opening in a brand new centre for women students, a centre founded by an American woman, a Mrs Anderson. It had one hundred students rooms and was called the Foyer International des Etudiantes. They telegraphed Dr Burnet saying there was an opening and, without even consulting me, he reserved a room for me. He was about to leave for Geneva to take up a new position there but, luckily, his wife was staying on a few weeks and would join him later. It meant that I could travel to France with her just before the university classes commenced in October. People in our strict family began to say that my mother had gone crazy. I had one uncle whom I thought I could count on because he had studied in France. He joined the other, saying, 'Your mother is crazy; she is sending you off to a city of perdition.'

"I began to prepare my departure. On the day I was to leave, one of my mother's brothers was to send his car to take me to the port and the boat for France. A family meeting was called with my uncle Tahar Ben Amar and the husband of an aunt who was our legal guardian, and an Islamic cleric. This was necessary, of course. Here was this young girl, an orphan, who wanted to go off to France to study on her own. As I was waiting for the car, I saw another one arriving. In it was the cleric, my two uncles and a cousin who was just a bit older than I. As he brushed passed me he whispered in my ear, 'You know, everybody knows, you aren't to be allowed to leave.'

"My aunt told my mother to cover herself and run to receive these men. My mother replied, 'Have them go upstairs, these aren't the first men or the last men that I will see.'

"So there we were, on the first floor in a sitting-room with our male guests, while the other women, my aunts, grandmother and sisters were all out of sight downstairs. Discussion, arguments, discussion – and in the meantime the car had arrived to take me to the port. I managed to tell the driver not to leave without me, no matter who told him to go away. And the discussions continued, slowly, slowly. 'How can a young girl who has never even been out of the city of Tunis' – I knew a bit of the city but not really even that much – 'be permitted to go so far away?' Mother answered simply that many people travelled, for pleasure or for health treatment, and that it wasn't such a big thing. She added, 'My daughter wants to learn, to study and you know that in Islam it is an obligation for both men *and women* to learn and improve themselves.' The cleric became silent. Finally one of my uncles said, 'Well, then she can leave *next* week because a young girl should only travel with her father, a maternal uncle or a brother.' Again my mother replied. 'She is leaving with a woman of whom I am as confident as my own self.' At this point I put on my coat and ran downstairs to the car because I knew we were about to miss the boat. In fact, the boat sailed a few minutes late that day because of me.

"The crossing was terrible, there was a storm and I was sick.

We quickly boarded a train to Paris and I arrived in what I thought was paradise. An extraordinary world. The student centre was beautiful. It was luxurious, furnished with lovely things, with great taste. Of the 100 students, there were 25 different nationalities and only about twenty French students. In those first years of study I became very friendly with an American student with whom I still correspond and with a Czech. There was only one other Muslim student, a Yugoslav girl whose father was a lawyer.

"I returned each year to Tunisia for a family visit. I remained in the student center for three or four years but then had to leave because they needed the rooms for newly arrived students. It was then that I had another stroke of luck because the Burnets had moved to Paris. I went to live with them and there, of course, I met a whole other world of scientists, writers and medical personalities. I was named an Externe des Hôpitaux de Paris. Dr Burnet had introduced me to his friends and thus I worked under some of the greatest doctors of the time. I was able to learn the latest techniques and theories. It was in this milieu that I finished my studies. I was with them for three years and as luck would have it, just as I finished my studies and went back to Tunisia, Dr Burnet was named Director of the Pasteur Institute in Tunis, so there we were, all together again. That was 1936. I had become almost an adopted daughter. Three people made it possible for me to study: my mother, and Dr and Mme Burnet. But without mother, I would never have been allowed to leave.

"When I came back to Tunisia I set up a private practice. I didn't even try to enter a hospital service. Since it was all controlled by the French, it would have been useless for me to try. There were several French women doctors in Tunis' hospitals at the time, but certainly no opportunity for a Tunisian woman. I set up a general practice. That is what intrigued me. Whether a woman, man or child, I liked diagnosing illnesses. But obviously, I was a curiosity for Tunisian women. At that point all women were veiled in Tunisia, for example. I never veiled. Women came to consult me about their gynaecological problems because the customs of the time made it virtually impossible for a woman to consult a male doctor about reproductive health. Only when they were very very ill did the shame make no difference. That is how I chose the specialty of gynaecology. I studied and then worked in gynaecological clinics to be able to prepare the exams for the specialty. Women consulted me on just about any problem they might have. Family disputes, relationships, child care and up-bringing and husband-wife problems. They would confide in me and, often, the subject of the number of children they desired would arise.

"In 1961, I was invited by the IPPF to go to Brighton; it was there that I met Dr Nazar, a young doctor who worked in Jerusalem and who stayed there until the troubles of 1967. Totally by chance I also visited East Pakistan, Dacca, in 1960–61. The Tunisian Women's Union had received an invitation and although I was not a member, they asked if I would go and represent them. I had also gone to New York to work in a family planning clinic there, to learn what was being done. As soon as contraceptives were allowed in Tunisia, in 1963, I started a family planning service at Charles Nicole Hospital where I was Head of the Gynaecological department. Two of three hospitals created family planning services in that period. Women learned about the contraceptive services by word of mouth very quickly. They were supposed to have the permission of their husband, of course. There were some husbands, for example, who would have the loop removed if they were going on a trip and leaving the wife alone. I witnessed that many times – and that practice still exists today.

"President Bourguiba had well prepared us for family planning. He was a leader in women's rights. He had abolished polygamy, had created a legal basis for women's rights in Tunisian law which, by the way, gave women the right to ask for a divorce. He was very advanced for his time not only in North Africa, but across the Arab world and Africa. Without Bourguiba, there wouldn't have been the progress there has been in Tunisia. His work for the status of women, his willingness to modernize Islamic interpretations, to forbid polygamy – all that was very important. And, of course, when you raise the status of women, you increase the willingness to limit the number of births in a family. Family planning became an open subject; people came without shame or controversy. There was no religious objection to family planning; it was seen as a health benefit for women who had five or more children, who were in poor health. When abortion became legal in 1965, I started placing intra-uterine devices immediately following the abortion. It worked very well. Many criticized us saying there would be problems but, in fact, I published a study of one thousand women which demonstrated that there was no haemorrhaging, rejection or infection.

"In 1968, several of us started the Clinic du Mont Fleury, the first clinic of the Tunisian Family Planning Association.

It became known as a model clinic throughout North Africa. Doctors came for training in family planning from all over sub-Saharan Africa – from just about all French-speaking countries. We even began a weekly consultation for husbands; we told women to send their husbands so that we could explain the advantages of family planning. It was there that we performed the first vasectomy. The clinic was funded by IPPF and funds from the German family planning services.

"I became the Director of the National Office for Family Planning, the government agency, for a year or so in 1970. The Minister of Health asked if I would take over the administration of the government agency. But I didn't want to be an office-bound administrator. I wanted to get back to treating patients. After a year I told M. M'Zali that I wanted to go back to my hospital work. I never wanted to be anything else than a doctor. Just that once I went into Government, but in fact, I only wanted to do my hospital work. I was asked to go into politics and always refused. When necessary, of course, one gets political. During the independence struggle I was vice President of the Tunisian Red Crescent (Islamic Red Cross). In 1952 the French army had stormed a village in the Cap Bon, destroyed homes, killed and raped the inhabitants. I went there, wrote a report and presented it to the French authorities.

"On a personal level, as a young woman doctor trained abroad, I think I was a bit frightening to young Tunisian men who might otherwise have courted me. Young men didn't dare show interest in me. I really didn't have time to think about it until such time as a Prince Charming came along and asked for my hand in marriage. He had been a classmate of my brother and had studied in Paris. He was a dentist and very handsome. He asked me to marry him; I hesitated for a time and then agreed. We had three children. Unfortunately he died in 1963 when my children were still in secondary school.

"None of my children wanted to be a doctor. My daughter is an archaeologist; one son is a dentist and the other a veterinarian. They used to say, 'Mother, we saw how much you worked, how often you were absent, that medicine was too demanding.' When I would arrive home and say I had to go back out to see a patient they would say, 'You are going again? Can't you stay home a while?' But I was always on call. I think that they just didn't want to live that way or, perhaps, there was not the vocation for medicine, I don't know. It was a difficult time for me, being a single parent with such professional responsibilities. Yes, it was very difficult."

Dr Christopher Luleka Anicet

Dr Anicet was born in Zaire. Following study in the Soviet Union, he sought a French-speaking country where he could pursue his specialized studies. He is now settled permanently in Tunisia.

"I first met Dr Ben Sheikh in her hospital wards. I had studied medicine in Kiev, and wanted to specialize in gynaecology. I applied to the University in Algiers, but didn't get an answer so I came to Tunisia in February 1969. I didn't understand much at all about French medical methods at that point. I needed a great deal of help. And it was Dr Ben Sheikh who gave it to me. Thanks to her I soon caught on to French methods. I had no intention of staying in Tunisia; I wanted to gain specialized training and move on. Again, thanks to Dr Ben Sheikh, I settled here.

"What was fascinating about her work, and learning from her, was her methodical, organized way of teaching and working. She was also very demanding. The files had to be just so, observations organized, well-reasoned and conclusions elucidated. I felt appreciated working with her. There was a lot of work and when she asked if I would take extra duty assignments, of course I did. She'd call up and say, 'Little one, I need someone in the ward right away.' I'd say OK and off I went.

"It is well known that Mme Ben Sheikh trained the best gynaecologists of Tunisia. For example, the aspiration technique for abortions: in other hospitals, only the Directors of departments would do them, not the residents or assistants. Mme Ben Sheikh made us do them. In fact her department was the first to do aspirations in Tunisia, she had brought back the technique from Hungary in 1970 when she went there for a conference. In the beginning everyone was against it, but we had no problems. It was the same with all the new technical breakthroughs or with caesarean sections. She wanted us to learn but she insisted that caesareans be done only as a last resort. She watched us for months before trusting us but when she did, then we were not only allowed, but required to perform all kinds of interventions done in her department."

Dr Chakroun, a native of Algeria, studied medicine in Paris, as had Dr Ben Sheikh. Married to a Tunisian, she lives permanently in Tunisia.

Dr Aicha Chakroun

"I'm a perfect example of the international contingent of Dr Ben Sheikh. She has always attracted people from other cultures and nationalities, who enjoy working with her. There have been a Russian woman, a Polish woman, French, Tunisians and Africans. I think she had a international bent, she liked foreigners and joked with them and developed very strong bonds of friendship with those who studied under her.

"I met her when I came back from France. I wanted to work in social services, with handicapped patients and in family planning. I was sent to see her by the Health Ministry. She said she would willingly teach me but that she had very few doctors and needed help in the gynaecological wards. For me, there was a mixture of fear, admiration, the aura of the first Tunisian or North African woman doctor – so well-known and respected. For me she was a great lady – with a capital L. Here I was, also a woman doctor, a colleague, an admirer of hers and now she was my boss. All this resulted in apprehension to serve her well.

"I became part of her team, in her hospital department. How lucky I was. I know others who came back at the same time as I and who worked with other gynaecologists. I don't mean to flatter myself, but I believe I am far better trained than they, due solely to the methodology and expertise of Dr Ben Sheikh. That said, we worked all the time. There was no such thing as fixed hours. If she called, if there was an emergency, we couldn't refuse. She was so generous of herself, how could we refuse her? She had a way of giving us pride in our work and what we were doing for Tunisian society. We worked hard for her, convinced that we were working for the benefit and health of women, of mothers and of children.

"In addition, Mme Ben Sheikh had a special quality that one didn't often find among French-trained Department heads. Most of them took advantage of their position to perform all the difficult interventions, to render themselves indispensable. But Mme Ben Sheikh had confidence in us young doctors; she was constantly there, yes, but she let us do the work. She let the young learn by doing and it worked wonders. When she was convinced someone was fully competent, she let them take over. She was, for example, the first woman who agreed to take on the responsibility of training gynaecologists and obstetricians. In other departments, the young had little chance to learn or better still, to learn by doing. So those who really wanted to work, could and in addition we were backed up by a Chief who said that she guaranteed our work. That kind of confidence in others is rare.

"For me Mme Ben Sheikh was not only the first woman doctor to have dared to go against social conventions, to study abroad, and to thus open up opportunities to other women; but she went far beyond that, convinced that she had to work for the well-being of women and, through that, for the entire family. It wasn't an easy life for her. She was widowed when the children were still young, and she had a terribly busy professional life – but one thing she taught us, beyond the rigour of our profession, was to take advantage of moments of joy and laughter. That was a principle of hers: to be able to laugh like a child when the situation gave us the opportunity.

"In the beginning, family planning was uniquely preventative. Slowly, with the evolution of the laws in Tunisia, it became curative. In 1973, abortion was legalized for those who had already had four children. Mme Ben Sheikh had understood the distress of women and believed that she should be ahead of the legal evolution. She considered the whole socio-economic situation of the family, the psychological situation of the woman. We had performed abortions prior to three months of pregnancy after the fourth child. She found herself confronted with situations that needed assistance for a host of reasons, which were not found in the laws of the time. For example, a woman whose husband worked abroad and who had become pregnant. In a society like ours, it was important to avoid scandal. You have to solve these personal and social dramas quickly and effectively. There is also the problem of unwed mothers. She allowed them to come into her ward and have their babies, which would then be put up for adoption; others wanted early abortions and still others who had come later, needed second trimester abortions which were performed with the utmost care, to the point where there were many medical articles published on this.

"Thanks to this, family dramas were avoided, cases of infanticide avoided. This was done by Mme Ben Sheikh, and our team participated in full confidence of her protection, outside the law. She was leading the law into a more liberal stance and she was able to do this because she never accepted a cent; she did it for the good of the family and the woman, never for personal gain. It was done in the hospital and without charge.

"Another factor in working with Mme Ben Sheikh was that of always working in an atmosphere of good humour and camaraderie. We were sure that we had a Chief who was supervising our work, who understood us, but someone who appreciated us for who we were and the way we worked. She respected us on the professional level but personally as well. For me, as a woman, it was very important to have this kind of support and from a woman who was of the avant-garde, who dared challenge laws. She would go to the courts, if necessary, to defend women's rights to give birth when and if they wanted, to have happy pregnancies, to give women the right to govern their lives and bodies. She never needed to defend these rights in a court but we knew by her attitude that she would not hesitate a minute to do so. No one ever dared to challenge her since she had an aura of being the first woman doctor who worked within her society for the welfare of women and families.

"The case of hymen repair is an example. It is part of the issue of how women are accepted in a society in transition. I remember being amazed by the situation of women when I came here and started working in Tunisian hospitals. Here we are in an Islamic society open to the winds of change. You found young women who were illiterate and closed to all notions of a changing society. They simply accepted anything society expected of them in closed family traditions. At the other extreme, you encountered the young Tunisian girl who had opened her mind and body to a Swedish style of liberty. Tunisian society was in total transition: it had opened up to Europe and begun to educate its female population. Yet in a traditional society, neither men nor women were ready to meet this transformation.

"Young girls thought they had found a Prince Charming and then found themselves alone, having 'lost' their virginity. And virginity was, of course, considered the principal element of a woman's worth, for her acceptance by society, or a husband. But to be married, one had to prove virginity on the wedding night. If not a virgin, the girl faced scandal, shame and a bleak future. Husbands would divorce girls who did not bleed, send them home in shame. The young girls were terrified at the thought of not being able to prove their virginity. But in whom could they confide? That is how they came to confide in a great woman, Mme Ben Sheikh. It was then that Dr Ben Sheikh realized that, in good conscience, 'Why shouldn't I try to help these young women? I'll repair the hymen three or four days before the wedding, in the hospital. It doesn't take more then ten or fifteen minutes. The girl then goes home, gets married, and there it was: a nightgown spotted with blood.' This wasn't done to cheat anyone, but to give young women a chance in life, women who were victims of a social transformation far beyond their control. We did this believing that we had a small role to play in the social transformation of the country and in the lives of young women.

"That was one of the contributions of Dr Ben Sheikh. She is a Tunisian through and through, and proud of it. She understood the problems of the people of her country. Her work was not just medical, on the contrary, she was totally attuned to social issues. She listened to women, to their joys, their fears, their anxieties and thus was able to stake out a role for her entire team, a role in the social aspect of medicine. And we followed her with pride. All of us learned this from her; without saying a word about her intent, she changed our vision of our role of doctors. We began to see the psychological and social side of our work.

"Mme Ben Sheikh is a very modest person. She never wanted to be visible or famous. Because of that, few understand the dimensions of her contribution to Tunisian society. Those of us who know her work hope that it will be made known to others for she was not just a medical doctor, she was a woman who marked her generation profoundly and, through those she taught, has influenced future generations as well."

Dr Tewhida Ben Sheikh

1909	Born Tunis, Tunisia
1928	Received Secondary school baccalauréat degree
1929	Left Tunisia for medical studies in France
1936	Received Medical Degree from University of Paris
1961	Attended IPPF meeting in Brighton, England
1963	Offered family planning services at Charles Nicole Hospital, Tunis
1968	Created the Clinic du Mont Fleury, first clinic of the Tunisian Family Planning Association
1970–71	Director of the National Office of Family Planning

Chapter 9
Professor Mohamed Ibrahim
(1911–1989)

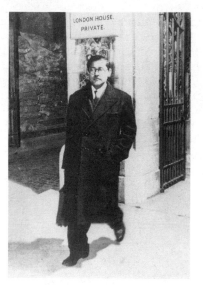

Dr Mohamed Ibrahim during his studies at the Royal College of Physicians, London, 1948.

Discipline is life

The land of Bengal is rich in history, art and literature. Conquered by Muslims in the 11th century, by the British in the mid-18th century and partitioned from India in 1947, the land of Tagore seceded from Pakistan to become a sovereign state barely 20 years ago. With 737 people per km², Bangladesh is one of the most populous nations of the world and one of the poorest. Its 115 million people live in an area 1/65th that of the United States, which has a population of 252 million. Sixty per cent of Bangladeshis are landless or marginal farmers.[1] It is a land where female literacy is 42 per cent that of males, where only 5 per cent of births are attended by health personnel and where female infant mortality is far higher than that for boys.[2] It is a land where 90 per cent of all girls are married before the age of 18.

It was in this context that a young woman doctor, Humaira Sayeed, introduced family planning to Bangladesh in the early 1950s. Witnessing the tragic results of an increasing number of non-medical abortions, Dr Sayeed sought the co-operation of doctors, lawyers and lay persons as co-founders of the Family Planning Association of Bangladesh in 1953. Barely four years later, Dr Sayeed died from complications of hepatitis. Among the friends she had brought into the association was Dr Mohamed Ibrahim, then Professor of Medicine at Dhaka Medical College. As a founder member of the Association and later Adviser to the President in charge of the Ministry of Health and Population Control, Labour and Manpower, Dr Ibrahim was an influential figure in expanding the planned parenthood services in Bangladesh. Based on his concern for quality training, the National Institute for Population Research and Training was created.

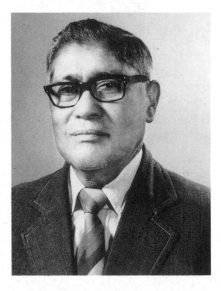

Dr Mohamed Ibrahim, co-founder of the Family Planning Association of Bangladesh and founder of the Bangladesh Institute of Research and Rehabilitation in Diabetes, Endocrine and Metabolic Disorder (BIRDEM) circa 1975.

Professor Ibrahim is best known, however, for his work in the treatment of diabetes. As the founder and president of the Bangladesh Institute for Research and Rehabilitation in Diabetes, Endocrine and Metabolic Disorders (BIRDEM) he demonstrated the importance of the treatment of diabetes in poor nations.

He was born into the family of a village postmaster in Murshidabad (now India) and had to walk several miles to school. Encouraged by his father to seek a higher education, he earned one of the few scholarships given to Muslim boys at the time. He remained a man of simple tastes, spurning a lucrative practice in the pursuit of improving medical care for the disadvantaged. Although his leadership of Bangladesh's national family programme was fairly brief, the innovations he introduced are credited with hastening the acceptance of family planning in circles resistant to the discussion or practice of planned parenthood. Dr Ibrahim never retired, but worked at BIRDEM until his death.

Mr Abul Hussein

As a young man, Abul Hussein had been a patient of Professor Ibrahim. A writer and poet who worked in the Ministry of Information, Mr Hussein served on the executive committee of the family planning association on behalf of the Ministry. Years later when the Professor became head of population programmes, he asked Mr. Hussein to join him. When the Professor left government, again Mr Hussein was asked to assist him, this time in the administration of BIRDEM where he now holds the post of Co-ordinator.

"Dr Ibrahim felt that anyone who came in contact with him was somewhat like his own child or relation. It was not friendship; it was something more than that. In our culture, someone who is a blood relation is more akin to you than anybody else. Whether people were related to him, whether he knew them or not, Dr Ibrahim would make them feel that they were one of his own family. The basis of his treatment was always empathy. Not sympathy, empathy. There is a great difference between the two words. Nobody had talked about this difference before Dr Ibrahim. I haven't heard this word uttered by any physician, social worker or scientist.

"Dr Ibrahim was concerned with the total person, that is why he was so interested in family planning: because maternity is so much a part of the total woman's life. His involvement in family planning started really with maternity care. As a professor of medicine, he found that among the pregnant women who came to him for treatment, many suffered from a haemoglobin count so low that they would have great difficulty bearing a child. Many would not survive. Family planning was necessary to saving mothers lives.

"In the early 1950s Dr Humaira Sayeed, a gynaecologist, was the motivating factor in introducing family planning here. She initiated the creation of the Family Planning Association. Dr Ibrahim and several other prominent individuals joined her. The government had been thinking about a population programme, but the creation of the Family Planning Association of Bangladesh (FPAB) was a key factor in influencing the government to act. In the beginning the family planning programme was part of the Ministry of Health. But because of the awareness created by FPAB the government came to feel that famiy planning was important as part of population control. The population growth rate was, I think, about 3.6 per cent at that stage. Prior to Dr Ibrahim taking over the Ministry of Health and Population Control, the programme was mostly clinically focused. It was a health programme, purely a doctors' programme. Doctors emphasized sterilization, tubal ligation. There were no motivation efforts. Dr Ibrahim started a multi-sectoral approach.

"Instead of it being a purely medical effort – or a health programme – Dr Ibrahim believed that success was dependent upon the involvement of other ministries as well. The Ministry of Social Affairs, of Education, the Planning Commission, the Ministry of Social Welfare and Youth, even the Labour sector were involved in the programme. They all joined in the motivation programme. The Labour Ministry, for example, would actually go to the factories and motivate workers about family planning. Each ministry set up a population unit. We worked with the Women's Affairs Ministry and with non-governmental organizations which worked with women.

"The Ministry of Religious Affairs was also a very important component in a country like Bangladesh, a very religious Muslim country. We began to work with the imams of the mosques and with the teachers in religious institutions like the Madrassah. In the rural areas religious leaders have tremendous influence on the people, tremendous. The people follow them more than other teachers. We used to train them, hoping that they, in turn, would motivate the rural people. The training consisted of seminars, orientation courses; we talked about women's health, the issue of family economics – more children than you could afford, children's health. We also talked about the teachings of the Koran. In the Koran there are mentions of *ajar*, the withdrawal method. It is authorized by the Koran.

"Initially we encountered – and it is still there to some extent – a bit of opposition from the religious groups. To counter that we took on an education programme. I took a group of 20 ullamas, religious leaders, to Indonesia and then to Malaysia. We toured the two countries for a month. We visited family planning clinics and showed them what family planning in a Muslim country was like. They debated the pros and cons of family planning with the Indonesian ullamas. When they came back to Bangladesh, although they did not come out and say these things, privately they told their students and disciples, 'It is absolutely necessary for us to take to family planning.'

"In the rural areas, couples do not talk about intimate things like how many children they will have. It is extremely difficult for the wife to speak up in such a male dominated society. The woman must take on whatever the husband gives to her. All decisions are taken by the man. When I used to visit rural areas and go to houses I would ask women if they were using family planning. They would say 'No, they don't know about it, nobody came to tell them about it'. We were working in the area; the family planning workers said that some of the women had IUDs, that many were planning. Later in the day, when the husband was no longer around, some of the women came to me to say 'These people came to us, gave us the services, we are using them but I couldn't tell you before because my husband was there and I don't want him to know. If he knew, he would be very angry.'

"We have family-life education in primary and secondary school but it is approached in a subtle way. . . . When you are planting coconuts you have to have a distance of some 20 feet between trees. If you don't, if they are closer, you will find that the fruit the tree bears will be smaller, not as healthy as if they were well-spaced. *Small family, happy family* was the motto of the FPAB. We have a family planning unit here at BIRDEM. We see some 40 to 50 peoples a day, all diabetic.

"I'm not a doctor. But Dr Ibrahim took me from the Ministry of Information. I have been the managing director of the Film Development Corporation, in radio and in television. I have experience in almost all the facets of the media so he took me to the Ministry to start a programme with emphasis on Information, Education and Communication. We didn't say 'communication' we said 'motivation'. So I was the first IEC consultant in the ministry. The radio is still used for motivation programmes; we have the tremendous advantage of being homogenous, one language, one religion; these are very important advantages. It was much easier to work here; unfortunately we have not achieved as much as some of the countries of South Asia which started their population programmes much later. There is no lack of services anywhere – but it is the follow up which is lacking. Motivation is needed not only among the clients but among the personnel as well. In the rural area we have nearly 50,000 FP workers; in every ward of the rural area there three are FP workers, in every union there is an FP assistant. But the workers in rural areas are not doing what is required, not doing the proper follow-up.

"Dr Ibrahim was a very great man, a man of varied interests. Many people know him today as a diabetologist and the founder of the Diabetic Association of Bangladesh and BIRDEM, this institute which is recognized all over the world as one of the finest institutions. Dr Ibrahim was never trained to be a specialist in diabetes. He was trained by the Royal College of Physicians, he worked for a while in tuberculosis and when he came back here he truly expected to be able to put his knowledge to good use. But the TB programme had not started at that stage; it was not well organized so he started working on diabetics. He started as a teacher in the medical college here, as professor of medicine.

"In 1946 the life expectancy was only 23 years. Endemic diseases – diarrhoeal, cholera, malaria – were very prevalent here. With the help of the World Health Organization and other agencies, many of these diseases are now well controlled. Dr Ibrahim perceived that if epidemic diseases were controlled, life expectancy of the people would rise; the long term diseases like diabetes, heart disease, hypertension, cancer would thus increase. His interest turned to the diseases which need life-long treatment. Once you have one of those diseases, you are going to live with them your entire life and the entire spectrum changes. The relationship between the doctor and the patient changes because you will now have to go to the doctor over and over again, all your life. You will have to keep your disease in check all your life. And once you can control it, you can lead a normal life for many years. Dr Ibrahim's interest in diabetes grew out of this. It is a life-long disease that has to be controlled. Based on that, in 1956 he started the Diabetic Association of Bangladesh. He brought succour, thus, to thousands of people in this country."

Dr Azad Khan

During the last years of Professor Ibrahim's life Dr Azad Khan, his son-in-law, lived with him in the family home in Dhaka. As a consulting doctor in gastro-enterology at BIRDEM, Dr Khan's opportunity to understand the personality and motivation of the Professor went beyond the family to the entire range of his professional and volunteer activities.

"There are several qualities that made Dr Ibrahim a very exceptional man. The first was his total commitment to whatever he did. This commitment meant of everything – his own health, wealth, his family – everything.

"I have never yet to meet a man with such vision. If he were born in a developed society, I'm sure he would have been much more famous because what he could visualize what it took others 15–20 years, even 30 years, to think was important.

In his early career he understood that medical care is not purely a medical matter. This is accepted now, but that was not so in the early 1950s, especially in the developing countries where one thought that medical care was something to do only with doctors. He said, 'That is not true, medical care is part of social care.' He realized that for life-long diseases, like diabetes, in a developing country where there is no social security or assured medical care, there has to be something like the Diabetic Association which looks after people, irrespective of the financial, social or educational status. He had vision about the question of family planning. He understood early on that the population question was going to become one of the top problems of Bangladesh. He was a deeply religious man, but he promoted planned parenthood very early. He was convinced about the need a long time back, before many other people here in this country.

"Since I had the opportunity of being with him most of the time, I was the person who often quarrelled, or argued, with him. For example he would say to staff at the hospital, 'Get this, or buy that' and they didn't dare say, 'But there is no money.' So I would be the one to say, 'We can't do it because we lack money.' He would look at me and say, 'Nothing has remained unaccomplished because of lack of finance.'

"When I thought about him after his death I wondered how he could possibly have accomplished so much. Then I thought a possible explanation was that he was indeed a megalomaniac. No rational person would be able to accomplish these things thinking rationally. He thought his power was really unlimited, that he could persuade people. Once he was convinced that something could be done, he would get it done. It is very difficult to summarize his influence on other people. After seeing what he had done I began to realize how much it was possible to accomplish in developing countries. It is the question of commitment, that I learned from him.

"His other influence on me was to teach me to visualize, to see what should be done and take people into your confidence. To organize medical care you must involve the patients, the incumbents, the people of the society. You have to involve the planners, the executives. It is this concept that would have taken a long time for people here to accept or understand.

"He never compromised his principles. I used to tell him that most of the doctors of his time were successful, wealthy practitioners and he could have been as well. He never had any money in the bank, no bank balance. When I married his daughter he didn't have enough money for the wedding; he had to borrow from his pension fund to be able to give her a proper wedding.

"He lived very humbly, modestly. His house was humble. He was a contented man; in fact I never saw him dissatisfied. Since he was a deeply religious person, whenever he had a failure, he thought that there might be something good in it and that success would come.

"For him there was no separation between family and work. His commitment was to life – a total commitment – so all parts of his life were one. It was the same as for a diabetic patient. He believed the patient's family was all part of the patient's situation and thus his cure.

"When he was called to act as an Adviser to the Prime Minister at a crucial time for Bangladesh, he was a bit hesitant to do so but once he was convinced that this was something demanded of him, that he would be in charge of family planning, he accepted. I think it is fair to say that his contribution was making family planning widely known. Making it popular to people. In developing countries people are shy when discussing family planning, with children, with each other, but these things can be discussed quite easily in a medical context. There is nothing indecent about it. I think it was Dr Ibrahim who made it possible. Yet it was quite unusual for a man like him, who was so religious, to discuss family planning openly with young children, talking about their puberty and all in decent language. He toured the entire country discussing family planning; it was part of his total commitment to everything he did.

"He became convinced that it was possible to achieve zero population growth. He had the idea of taking a particular area of the country and proving that one could achieve zero population, there in that area, as an example to the entire country. I don't know if he had stayed in the position for longer if he would have achieved it. But he wanted to show the country that it could be done. He thought if he could manage the programme for five years he would be able to achieve it.

"He left his position as Adviser to the government because he did not want to join in the political fray. It was not 'his place' to join a political party. The President had a great deal of respect for him. When he finally told him that he had to resign, the President took his hand and put it on his heart – the President called him *sir* out of respect – 'Sir, I am in pain because you are leaving but the situation in the country demands that it has to be a political post.'"

Mahnur Rahman

As a graduate in social work from the University of Karachi, Mahnur Rahman pursued nutrition studies and eventually became the Director of Training at the National Institute of Population Research and Training (NIPORT) where she currently works. She has been a volunteer for the Family Planning Association of Bangladesh since 1967.

"I first met Professor Ibrahim in 1958, when he was the president of the Diabetic Association. I was a student on job training for social work. We were assigned to go to the Diabetic Association to observe its organization, record-keeping and follow-up system.

"Eventually I had an opportunity to work under his guidance from 1976–79. He was then Advisor at the Ministry of Health and Family Planning. I was Project Director of a Health Nutrition and FP Education Project. He considered me one of his dearest ones because of my involvement in the nutrition project and what I was able to accomplish there.

"I once asked him how he became interested in family planning. He told me, 'Humaira Sayeed used to call me and invite me to the meetings, saying she needed my advice and guidance.' But having worked with Dr Ibrahim I truly believe that he wanted to help women avoid undesired pregnancies.

"There is practically no sex education within families here. Young girls go to marriage without knowing anything about their bodies or about sexuality. Even the issue of menstruation is kept from them. Family planning was never actually prevented, that is true, but socially it was not accepted. I've heard that when they held the first meetings it was not reported in the papers. They were afraid of criticism if they publicized family planning activities.

"Dr Ibrahim was a dynamic leader. He was very firm about what he wanted to achieve – and would go ahead and do it. He was firm, he might appear frightening but when you knew him well you would see he was at heart a very gentle man. I will always remember him for his contribution to women's development in Bangladesh. He took a very bold step in 1976 by appointing 13,000 women to work in village family planning programmes. Due to some bureaucratic procedures, the appointment could not take place for a long time. But Professor Ibrahim gave orders to complete the appointment by 31 March 1976. To do this in 1976, when only 6 per cent of the women of Bangladesh were literate, was a miracle."

Mohamed Ibrahim

1911	Born Murshidabad, India
1940	Calcutta Medical College, receives a MB
1945-47	Resident Physician, Calcutta Medical College
1947-48	Civil Surgeon of Chittagong District
1948	Studied at the Royal College of Physicians, London receiving a MRCP
1953	Co-founder of the Family Planning Association of Bangladesh
1956	Founder of the Diabetic Association of Pakistan
1975-77	Adviser to the President, charged with the Ministry of Health and Population Control, Labour and Manpower and the Ministry of Social Welfare
1989	Died while still Director of Bangladesh Institute of Research and Rehabilitation in Diabetes, Endocrine and Metabolic Disorders (BIRDEM)

References

1. World Bank, Social Indicators of Development 1990, The Johns Hopkins University Press, Baltimore, p. 22
2. Ibid.

Chapter 10
Elsie Locke (b. 1912)

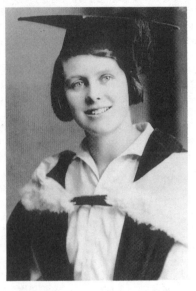

Elsie Farrelly upon her graduation from the University of Auckland in 1933, the first of her family to attend university.

All I can do is pull my oar in the ways available to me

Elsie Farrelly Locke was born barely 20 years after New Zealand became the first sovereign state to introduce women's suffrage (1893). A land settled by farming families from the British Isles, New Zealand had long relied on women's contributions to national life and well-being. Her life's work has helped document those contributions and expand women's rights and roles in New Zealand society. Author, peace and environmental activist, socialist, women's rights advocate and a mother of four, Elsie Locke is an historian of the social history of her country for the past half century. She is an activist who, when she feels her contribution is no longer needed, simply goes on to the next challenge. From advocating rights for the unemployed to the legalization of family planning, from environmental, anti-nuclear and peace movements to the rights of housewives and the promotion of natural childbirth, Elsie Locke's commitment to social justice is continuous. Her interest in Maori culture led her to study and become fluent in the Maori language, which then enabled her to contribute to a better understanding of Maori culture and history. She was awarded an honorary doctorate in 1987 for her ability to join scholarly work with social responsibility.

Born to a family of modest means, the young Elsie Farrelly worked her way through university during the great economic depression of the 1930s. The poverty she saw around her greatly influenced her thinking and resulted in her joining the Communist Party. At the time New Zealand was a nation of 1.5 million (1936). Isolated geographically, dependent on exporting a few products, New Zealanders viewed themselves as vulnerable to foreign powers, in particular Japan whose militarism during the 1930s cast fear over many Asian nations. Historian Mary Dobbie has described the times:

> For most New Zealand families the mid-thirties were anxious years, the Depression barely lifting, unemployment widespread, ill-health and over-crowded housing adding to the strain. Country folk, forced off their farms when mortgages foreclosed, moved in with relatives or squeezed themselves into run-down rooms along with the city unemployed, making worse an already desperate housing problem . . . The fear of underpopulation pervaded newspaper articles, church and political utterances. Members of the Government were hinting at the possibility of war and the need for men in the ranks. And women, listening to the admonitions from church and city fathers, believing that they did, indeed, hold the destiny of the country in their busy hands, but wondering guiltily how another pregnancy would be avoided.[1]

Reliance on illegal abortions was high; deaths from septic abortion were frequent, as were resulting chronic ailments. Mary Dobbie notes, "The Obstetrical Society was well aware of the high mortality from septic abortions; in 1934 out of a total of 118 maternal deaths, 42 were so caused, giving New Zealand one of the highest maternal death rates in the world. . . . Though aware that the greatest number of death occurred among married women with three, four, or five children, the Obstetrical Society seems to have avoided any consideration that contraception might offer a remedy."

It was in this climate that Elsie Locke and her companions began the struggle for the legalization and distribution of contraceptives.

Our conversation took place in 1991 in the small study – her office – of her house in Christchurch, where she and her husband recently celebrated their fiftieth wedding anniversary.

Elsie Locke

"The more I think about my mother, the more amazed I am, really. It's funny, the older you get the more you do. She never had any proper education. Her father was a bush worker, cutting timber. There was a lot of gold mining going on and they needed timber props for the mines. Her brothers took up the same work, and they worked over on the West Coast. My grandmother decided she would join the men but having had such a dreadful journey out from England in the first place, she swore she would never go by sea. She loaded the essential family goods onto a wagon and with the four youngest children just trekked over the pass. My mother was just a young girl at the time. She had to go into household service; it was the only available work. She hated it; she told me some very sad stories about service work. However, her mother took ill and was ill for about four years with some form of paralysis. She wasn't able to move much, probably stress, I would think. My mother and her sister cared for her. When she died, my mother went back into service again.

"So mother never had any opportunity for education. Neither did my father. He was an intelligent man, very poor at handling his business but certainly a very keen reader. So they met up, got married and had six children. I was the youngest. There was never a chance to improve herself or do anything like that. Furthermore, my father couldn't manage his business affairs at all – he was a builder and a very good craftsman – but he went bankrupt three times. So we were always up against it. As children we were dressed in clothes that relations sent us. Both my parents were very keen that we should have the education that they missed out on. Mother went to all sorts of trouble to see that we had opportunities. You wouldn't call her a feminist in the ordinary sense but she had her ideas, all right. One of the things she used to say to us four girls, 'There's nothing a man can do that a woman can't attempt. Give it a try'. She always said it was as good to be a woman as to be a man. Once when I was in my early teens and the boys were having a good time at the girls' expense, I said, 'Oh I wish I'd been a boy' and she said, 'No you don't, it's much better to be a woman.'

"She was a very generous woman; she didn't find fault with anybody except hypocrites. I remember saying to her when I was quite a small girl and being scolded for untidiness or spilling things, 'It will be nice to be grown-up; I won't do those things. I'll be good all the time.' She replied, 'Elsie you don't *know* the wicked things that grown-ups can get up to.' And my word, there was feeling in those words; I could tell she had been done wrong all right, there had been things that she never talked about.

"My father also grows in my estimation as time goes on. He was an estimable character in many ways: he never drank, smoked, gambled or went out with wild women. In fact he was a pillar of the temperance movement. We were all brought up strict teetotallers – the worst thing you could ever do was get drunk. But he had one fault, particularly when his finances were going wrong, he had a terrible raging temper which was really like temporary insanity. He'd rage and storm and swear and threaten. Normally he never swore. And Mum would stand with her back to the wall, literally, stand there quietly and let him storm away and never say anything. But this used to frighten us. And we'd say, 'Why don't you retaliate, why don't you say something?' Of course now I know that she was very careful not to provoke him. We'd just get out of the house and not come back for hours. We held that against Dad, really. We were always on Mum's side. but now I understand that it was something he couldn't help.

"Mum always had to manage the money; he didn't have to worry about that. But he never restricted us at all. He never said, 'You are not to try this' or 'You're not to do that.' We were given a lot of freedom to do things that were unusual at the time. You know there are so many parents who lay out their children's lives for them. But opportunities were not there for girls at the time. The puritan ethic simply made us know that 'girls aren't as good as boys' – put downs are a subtle sort of thing. Girls didn't believe much in themselves. They were told that they were to settle down and raise a family, that was the best things for them. It was their destiny. I got married and had a family but I never regarded it as the only thing in life.

"At the time, there was no sex education. This is the one place where my mother really failed. She must have had some terrible inhibitions because she didn't talk to us much at all. My first period was unexpected. I had heard some vague sort of story about 'sooner or later there will be blood in your pants' but that never meant anything to me. Mum didn't prepare me for it; she just told me how to deal with it. She made home-made towels and taught me to wash them and put them through the big boil later. That was all she taught me, to keep myself clean. The big shock about my period was that it was thought that it was wrong for a girl to go swimming – 'Hold on, wait a minute, you mean I have to give up swimming?' Dreadful. That is what affected me most. My sisters knew practically nothing when they got married, only what they picked up. But I was a little more cunning. When I was working in the University library, there was a medical library attached to it. The girl I was working with, who was in charge, was no older than me – and no better informed than me – so we just raided the medical library. We found all sorts of interesting things. It's curious, to be sure, but family planning came to be accepted *long before* sex education. Even now. It seems to me that's the wrong way around.

"My interest in family planning was a concern for those around me. It wasn't any particular political belief at the time or because of one personal experience; it was a whole weight of experiences. When I went to Wellington I got very involved in the unemployed movement. I had joined the Communist Party and since there was quite a shortage of active people I volunteered to work with the unemployed. In so doing I mixed with other women. We started a paper, called *Working Woman*. The idea of the paper was to interest women in being more active themselves. There were many women among the unemployed but that fact tended to be pushed aside. I believed a paper would be a good organizing medium. And it was. Out of it grew an organization called the Working Women's Movement. The interesting thing about it is that very few of those women were communists although they were selling and organizing around a communist paper. It was simply that nothing else was offered to them. I was very keen, and still am, on equal pay for equal work but through the journal I began to develop interest in other women's issues. I suppose I took them up one way or another all the time.

"Most of our readers were wives of the unemployed. The question of unwanted babies came up again and again. Another baby in those conditions was something awful, a desperate tragedy and they used to refer to 'getting rid of it'. So I started asking a few questions, 'What's this getting rid of it?' Well, there were needles and crochet hooks and jumping off things and all sorts of quack ideas rampant among them. It was awful, absolutely awful, they shouldn't be getting pregnant. My concern wasn't anything to do with morals or women's rights, it was simply – how are these poor desperate families going to avoid having another child that they can't feed?

"As you can imagine, birth control was a very controversial issue. There was the moral thing, you know, this information is going to get into the hands of the unmarried and the only people who should have sex are the married. So we were going to 'corrupt morals'. We were accused of encouraging bad girls in their bad ways. It would have been much better to encourage bad girls than to have all the other unhappy results of ignorance. . . . Some of the things that were said were very peculiar. I remember one that said women would stop having children if they had the opportunity to prevent them. It's really hilarious, isn't it. Look at the trouble people go to now, *in vitro* fertilization and all this kind of thing in order to have a child. I also learned that it was a tricky business mentioning birth control to a family who didn't have any children. So we had to think of family planning the other way as well: not only help people to plan births but put them in a position to have a family if they wanted one.

"There was also a lot of this idea 'Populate or perish'; doing your duty for the State: 'Lie back and think of England'. Have you heard that one? It was part of your duty. It was one of the things that was fed to you. Then of course there was a large religious section that thought you should never deny Nature's course. Particularly the Catholics, but there were others who thought that way, saying, 'God sends the babies, don't you try to stop them.'

"There was a great deal of prejudice but it wouldn't have extended to the Maori. The Maori population declined all last century; it was very low at the turn of the century. That was its lowest point, down to about 45,000 which is very small. The reasons have to do with the wars and the loss of land and the fact that when the Europeans' arrival occurs, as is the case for most all indigenous people, they pick up simple diseases like measles which kill them off. It is a very tragic story. But once the Maori population started to grow again, they were very keen that it should keep growing. I don't think birth control was the least bit of interest to Maori people at the time we started. And the average *pakeha*[2] didn't worry about it. Their villages were very remote and they hardly ever saw a white person. They lived very largely off their own resources. The Maori world was quite separate in fact until the wartime. It was then they were encouraged to come to the city in greater numbers to work. Today, the Maori population is largely urbanized and is using family planning. In fact they have their own family planning groups. It's due to the adaptations they had to make to urban living.

"I certainly got myself in a lot of arguments when we first started our family planning organization in Wellington. But somehow it never bothered me. I think, again, it is partly my mother's influence. She'd say, 'Stand up for yourself. If you think it's right, go for it.' She knew I was involved in family planning as part of the unemployed movement and she didn't mind. Funnily enough, in spite of her inhibitions she used to say 'Never be ashamed of the human body; it's the most beautiful thing in the world.'

"Women's knowledge was very poor. One of the things we did, including amateurs like me, was to talk to meetings with diagrams, showing how the reproductive system operated. People didn't know. They just knew that they slept with their husband and after nine months a baby came. But just *why* and *how* – the sperm meeting the egg and that business – was all new. It seems astounding now. There's been a lot of progress, even though there is still very little sex education in the schools. There has always been a lobby that says it is the parents' duty to educate their children. Of course the answer to that is – how often they *don't*. Children still get the wrong information from the wrong sources.

"My activism in family planning only lasted about four years, while I was in Wellington. Do you know the reason for the complicated title Sex Hygiene and Birth Regulation Society? It was to douse criticism as much as anything. Sex Hygiene really meant sex education and Birth Regulation meant that you were not trying to prevent anybody from having families – you just wanted to make it possible for children to be spaced. We took up the name family planning as soon as we realized this was the English name and a much better one.

"I came to Christchurch in 1941 when the war was on. I came to get married. Of course I was married before, but that fell to pieces. The Freeman marriage was a silly one, really. When I look back I wonder how I could have been so stupid. Fred Freeman was another communist; we got along well at the start but then it began to fall apart. I was very keen to have a baby but he wasn't. He said it would impede our political work. I finally talked him into it. But when the baby was halfway here, he made it obvious that this was a hindrance and he didn't want it. We rowed about it; I felt I was being done down. And there were other differences already anyway. So finally I said to him, 'It's my baby – it's *my* baby – You git; just leave it to me.' And of course I was too proud to accept any assistance. In any case he wasn't in a position to give any. I had no money whatever from him after the baby was four months old. So I had to resort to all sorts of ways to support him; it was a real struggle. But we got by. And he was a lovely baby. One of the things that attracted me to Jack (my husband for 49 years) was that every child is a delight for him. He's crazy on little kids, and still is as a grandfather. He loves the lot. It wouldn't matter a drat damn whose baby this was. So when I married him he got a three and a half year old boy, too.

"When I arrived in Christchurch, I had to settle into a whole new environment. With the war on, there were all sorts of things to be done. I wasn't in the best of health; I'd worn myself to bits. Family planning here was going like a charm. There were some very good people who were doing a very good job. So I didn't get involved. I got interested in other things – some of the problems affecting housewives during the war, rationing and the like. I've been involved with peace things regularly for a long time. I was always criticized by the Communist Party for pacifist tendencies – and feminist tendencies, for that matter. I was never happy supporting war.

"During World War II, of course, you couldn't do anything. But shortly after the war, all this business about the Cold War set in. Very quickly, fear of Russia and all that. We were touched by stupid McCarthyism as well. By 1949, only three years after the end of the war, they brought up peacetime conscription again. There was a big movement against that, but we didn't succeed. The Labour Party Conference and the Federation of Labour Conference were against conscription so the government decided to have a referendum to get around this opposition. All the forces of the state went into persuading people to vote yes – and they did. The logic was that we had to be ready to fight Russia. It's awful when you think of it. You just get over one war and then everybody is getting ready for the next. Then of course the Chinese went and had a revolution. More problems for those who feared them.

"I've been involved in campaigns like that ever since, but the one I was most involved with was the Campaign for Nuclear Disarmament. Our work paralleled others' work abroad; we were in touch with those in the US. We had our links with SANE and with British CND. We were involved in opposing nuclear tests in the Pacific as well; it was all part of a whole. If you look at the policies we advanced about 1960, nearly all have been won. New Zealand even took a resolution to the United Nations for a Nuclear Free Pacific. It was co-sponsored with Fiji. There were abstentions, of course, but no contrary votes at all. We got as far as that. Then the next government came in and stopped the whole thing.

"I came to the realization that we were destroying the earth by a rather strange experience. I had a long lie in hospital with TB of the spine. When I left Wellington in 1941, I had a tubercular gland in my neck. It was lanced and nothing showed up for a time although it had gotten into the bone. It began to show up toward the end of the war. It got worse and worse. But it was a long time before it was diagnosed as spinal TB. The symptoms were just pain, awful pain. Oh, dear. I had a bad back and the pain was appalling. Bone TB was not considered infectious in any way. It is not treated by drugs, but by immobilizing the joint completely for no less than two years. I was close to three years on the flat of my back, on a special bed, not moving my back at all. I could move my arms, legs and head but that was all. It sounds awful but as a matter of fact, to be honest, it was a life-saver for me because I had time to read, time to *think* and time to *observe* and I'm very grateful for it.

"I was very discontented about a lot of things in the Communist Party before I went in hospital. I couldn't sort out my thoughts because we all worked so hard. You just keep going and you don't have time to sit and think. I came out still prepared to be a Communist but wanting the Communist Party to take notice of some of my new thoughts. How ridiculous! While I was in hospital I started to read a bit about soil erosion. A few of our scientists began to point out what we have done to the land in this country and I've been interested ever since. I went so far as to write a pamphlet on it and offered it to the Communist Party. The reply was, 'The workers aren't interested in this'.

"I really got quite concerned about environmental degradation. I have a very strong feeling for my country and when I realize what we have done to it, I weep. European settlement has been cruel as far as the land, forests and wastes are concerned. Settlers go into a totally different environment without knowledge of how to treat it properly. In addition, they go in with the capitalist system which sets out to exploit it. Look at us here in New Zealand – the seals and the whales were first, then the forests; we used up our gold and cleaned out everything. I still have exactly the same feelings about the system we live under as I had when I first started. I just don't think the Communist Party went about it the right way to change it.

"We used to talk about women's rights. There was no talk about women as if they were almost a separate species – oppressed by men who were out to oppress them. The Communist Party wanted to get women in along with the men and any element of pointing out that women had separate interests wasn't welcome. I was actually placed in charge of work among women which is how I managed to get the paper going, saying, 'Well this is what we've got to do.' but the interest was more in what women could do in the unemployed movement. In the 1930s there was quite a wave of feminism. The support given to women today is a good indication of the breadth of the movement in the community at the time. Equal pay for equal work and the right of women to work. One of the things that happened in the depression was that married women were denied the right to work very often. Married women teachers were sacked in preference for single teachers and on and on. This stirred up a lot of interest.

"We've had three waves of feminism in New Zealand, one in the 1890s, when the fight was on for the vote for women. You must know that we were the first sovereign country in the world to introduce the right to vote. We were beaten to the draw by the state of Wyoming and hot on their heels was South Australia. But those were just states; we were the first sovereign country to introduce rights for women. The interesting thing to me is that almost everything that has been taken up by the modern women's liberation movement was foreshadowed by those women in the 1890s, including wages for wives. 'Don't have war pictures hanging on your walls', 'Don't educate your children for war' – all sorts of things, including equal pay. I've had a sort of fringe interest in the women's liberation movement. I haven't been particularly deeply involved but I'm regarded by most as a feminist. If feminism is 'up with the women and down with the men', I've always said that I am not that kind of feminist. I think liberation is for us all. We've got to get away from these old sexist ideas.

"I'm an incorrigible optimist. I've got a very biological approach to life. I just see us as part of the animal kingdom and animals do not give up life readily. We have to look at it collectively; we have to do something about our planet before we ruin it. there have been some positive developments recently. Ten years ago, who would have thought the world would be so concerned about environmental issues? In the long run we will get around to some sort of socialism, we can't avoid it. This system is just too exploitative both of natural resources and of people. And if we expect all the Third World people to go on being at the bottom of the heap forever, we've got another think coming.

"I'm strongly opposed to the 'right to life movement'. Every time they come out to picket and I get a chance, I go and tell them off. *They don't know what they are doing.* We want 'wanted babies' but we don't want a single one that is not wanted. Not on this over-crowded planet. The argument that family planning is going against the rights of people in Third World countries, or indigenous peoples, is seriously raised in left-wing circles and I've had to fight it. They say, 'This is imperialism trying to stop the poor from multiplying so we will come into our own'. It's a load of rubbish. And the men reinforce it, of course. It doesn't matter what culture it is, if a woman doesn't want any more children, it is her right to say no. It is a pure question of women's rights and women's health. The Catholics talk about *natural* family planning without thinking that it takes two to practice it. A woman may decide she wants abstinence but would her husband? That's doubtful. And let us not forget that a lot of men get drunk.

"I'm a straight-on person, in anything I do. I just went ahead and did whatever needed doing and found someone to help when necessary, I suppose. But there's a limit to what you can do. You have to let a lot of things go by that you feel badly about because you can't be active or intervening or speaking-up about everything. You'd be regarded as a total crank if you tried it. For me it was always what happened at the grassroots that counted. I never had any ambition to get into parliamentary politics.

"I grew up in the country where I had a wonderfully free childhood. I was never expected to be a conformist, so it was never any bother to me to be a non-conformist. The fact that we were hard up was quite irrelevant. Or at least, if anything, it taught me to accept simple things and a simple standard of living. We've never chased the flesh pots, we needed an adequate standard of living and worked to earn our little home. We never wanted much more, really, because we never needed it. So I think I was extraordinarily lucky. I didn't have a lot of self confidence for a lot of my life because I had a feeling that I was a bit of country bumpkin in the big city. But that was gone years ago. I don't give a damn about this now. I used to veer between no confidence at all, and loads of it. That's nothing. You get over that.

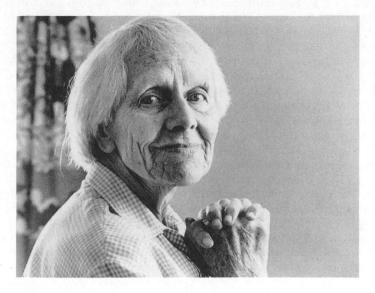

Elsie Farrelly Locke, historian, environmentalist, socialist and women's rights activist activist at her home in Christchurch, New Zealand in 1991.

"Right now I'm cleaning up the immense quantities of paper in this house so that if I die in the night my heirs and successors will not be driven to desperation. I've got some children's books that I'm anxious to finish. It is often said that the reason women have a longer life span than men is because they don't retire. To be honest, what I'd like to retire from is cooking. I hate it."

Janet Wilkinson Paul

Perched high on a hill near the Botanical Gardens in Wellington, Janet Paul's bungalow shares a garden with a shed-like painting studio. Her deceased husband was a publisher and bookshop owner; she is a typographer, layout designer and painter. The Pauls were the first to publish the works of Elsie Locke. Recently Janet Paul and Elsie Locke collaborated on a historical book about early New Zealand entitled *Mrs Hobson's Album*.

"I first heard of Elsie Locke through my husband. He often spoke of her as one of the younger university contemporaries whom he greatly admired. She came from quite a poor country home and had put herself through university. He was involved with the university paper and I think he came across Elsie as a writer. I didn't meet her until we were married and had our publishing house. It must have been in the late '50s. Elsie wrote to my husband and said she was writing a children's book, a historical reconstruction about a widow who settled in New Zealand with her children. We did indeed publish, *The Runaway Settlers*.

"She has some of the best qualities of the New Zealander who grew up in the depression in the thirties and through the experience gained a great sense of social responsibility. She is very fair minded, well informed and has a basic belief in the rights of everybody to good education, good housing and medical care. You see, all that is being eroded here. The government is trying to make us efficient but efficient isn't the same as caring for people. That thinking permeates her writing, even the children's novels which recount the social history of this country.

"She is an incredibly courageous person. If she wanted to support a cause, like family planning at a time when it was not 'the flavour of the month', she went ahead – or a pacifist, an active supporter of trade unions and the labour movement, an anti-nuclear activist when it came up – always caring about civil liberties. If Elsie thinks its the right thing to do, she'll just carry on and do it. She is a practical person as well. She was trained in history and therefore was able to work on children's books at a time when she could do little else. When you are crippled and have young children and not much money, school publications are an answer. In the '40s and '50s they were a very good market for writers. Quite a lot of our good writers wrote factual and scientific works for school journals for different grades, but for all the children in all the schools. Writing gave her a way of expressing her values, of influencing others.

"She learnt Maori a long time ago. Now not that many *pakeha* intellectuals set themselves to learn Maori out of sensitivity to their history. She attended lectures and studied. She can write Maori and correct Maori spelling when you get into problems. Her ability to communicate with Maori friends gives her an extra dimensions which few *pakeha* historians have.

"She is the epitome of the best kind of New Zealander of that period – who couldn't just sit back and let other people do things. She felt she had to do her part. It wasn't easy with three kids, so little money. She took a stand on the major social justice causes of her time and then, when they were well on track, she'd turn to the next cause, where she could be useful. That's the way she has kept going, I'm sure. Anything that requires her attention, she'll have a go at it."

Mary Woodward

During the 1960s and '70s the Campaign for Nuclear Disarmament was very active in New Zealand. A Quaker and peace activist, Mary Woodward worked closely with Elsie Locke in organizing those efforts. We talked one afternoon in her Auckland home.

"Elsie and I worked extremely well together in CND because we were very fond of one another and shared an enormous concern for our children. I think that was the principle feeling for both of us for doing anything – to think of our children, not just our kids but they represented all others as well – 'We just can't let these kids go up in smoke.' We had that same basic commitment and this stuck us together.

"She was an extremely good chairperson. The people who attacked us on the Campaign for Nuclear Disarmament were to the far-left. They attacked us for being too respectable, too bourgeois: 'You're sold out to middle class' and all that. I remember people getting into a terrible tizzy at a meeting in Wellington about that sort of thing and Elsie taking charge by saying, 'We are here to fight the bloody *bomb* and not to fight one another. And if you lot don't shut up I'm going to close this meeting and declare it out of order.' Elsie would never be phased by a difficult situation on the stage because she had been so well trained by her party work. She relied on answering calmly, with the facts, and on her own principles. She'd say, 'If you really believe in something you don't need to be angry about it to defend it. You simply have to state your case and explain why you believe in that way.' That's been the basis for everything Elsie has done, really. She has stuck to these very strong principles of concern for other people, for the integrity and dignity of other people.

"We constantly said that the nuclear deterrent doesn't make sense, for a common sense point of view. And, it's immoral. All this fuss about *abortion* – one life? my goodness me! Every nuclear test in the atmosphere destroys eggs and unborn children. The use of one nuclear bomb would maim unborn children as it still does in Hiroshima and Nagasaki. How can we possibly justify it and make all that fuss about a woman not being allowed to have an abortion because the unborn child is sacred? You can't have it both ways!

"When Elsie was involved in starting family planning, she was a member of the Communist Party. In the climate of the times, that was enough to damn everything you do. She was also involved with getting child care centres started. You can't have equal rights for women until you have adequate child care. Elsie knew the problem well. When her first husband left her, she was on her own and found it very difficult. She realized there was no adequate child care and yet she had to go to work to support herself and her child.

"Elsie became very ill with spinal TB and while she was on her back she read her way out of the Party. She had never had the time, before, to read and think.

"Elsie has had a significant influence on ordinary people. Her articles are written so that everyone can read them; her books are simply written. She gives a lot of radio talks, talking about everyday affairs, about the current economic mess, about foreign policy. She's also had a great influence on appreciation of Maori affairs because she puts it all so clearly and so kindly. Those who read her books can't help but have a better understanding of New Zealand history. She has been an inspiration to other people; she cheered us up."

Mary Dobbie

Journalist and historian Mary Dobbie lives in a cliffside house high above the Tansmanian Sea, not far from Auckland. Her fondness for Elsie Locke is based on both personal and professional experiences. As the author of *A Matter For Women, the New Zealand Family Planning Association 1936 – 1976*, she documented the work of the many individuals whose efforts led to the creation of the association. Among the anecdotes she told about Elsie Locke, the following is perhaps most revealing.

"In 1939, when Elsie was pregnant with her first child, she heard about a natural approach to childbirth developed by a famous British obstetrician. It was based on a series of exercises, the Margaret Morris exercises, and through her friends in British family planning, she obtained a book explaining the method. She wanted to try it. At her first appointment at the maternity hospital she took the book along and asked the physiotherapist if she would help her do the Morris method.

Unbeknown to Elsie, the physiotherapist was a total enthusiast of the method and Elsie was the first to inquire about it. Here at last was someone who would try it out. So they worked together, preparing Elsie for natural childbirth. When the time came to go into labour, all the midwives of the maternity hospital gathered around Elsie's bed to watch. Without need of medication of any kind she brought her baby to birth.

"She later told me that she had been confident she could do it, cope with the natural birth – but she had had no idea of the emotional elation that she experienced when she brought her baby to birth in that way. In the grey world of the depression years she had just come through, this was almost like a miracle, a wonderful experience that brightened everything for her."

Elsie Farrelly Locke

1912	Born Wiauku, New Zealand
1930–33	Auckland University, BA
1933–41	Wellington area, active in movements of the unemployed; founder and editor of *The Working Woman*
1936	Convened first meeting of the Sex Hygiene and Birth Regulation Society, becomes its Secretary
1941	Married Jack Locke, Christchurch. Several years of illness
1957–72	Active in New Zealand Campaign for Nuclear Disarmament and opposition to Vietnam War
1958	Wins Katherine Mansfield award for non-fiction essay in leading quarterly *Landfall*
1965–88	Publishes novels, essays, historical research
1987	Honorary degree of Doctorate of Literature, University of Canterbury

Reference

1. Mary Dobbie, *A Matter for Women, New Zealand Family Planning Association (1936 – 1976)*, unpublished manuscript
2. *Pakeha* – Maori word for European

Chapter 11
Dr M.A. Barnor (b. 1917)

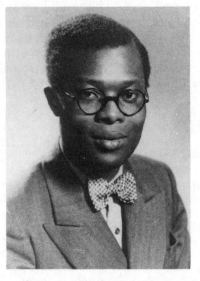

*M.A. Barnor during his studies at Edinburgh University,
circa 1948.*

*The traditional ways have changed completely. Before it was
the parents or the grandparents who taught children about
sexuality. Now the parents think that since the children go to
school, it is the school which should teach about these things.
The school thinks it should be the parents' responsibility. There
are so many attempts at abortion. It is tragic.*

Mrs. Peace Acolatse, midwife,
Peaceville clinic on the outskirts of Accra, 1991

Creating consensus and an organization

Modern Ghana is one of the most resource-rich nations of West
Africa. It was known to European traders as the Gold Coast,
and the land and its people were plundered for slaves and

gold from the 15th century on. In the beginning of the 19th century, much of modern Ghana was under the suzerainty of the Asante tribe with enclaves of British, Dutch and Danish trading interests which maintained forts and castles along the coast.[1] By 1874 the British consolidated their control of the Gold Coast by declaring it a British Crown Colony. In 1957 Ghana became the first British colony in Africa to become an independent nation. It is estimated that by 1940 the population of Ghana was approximately 3.23 million.[2] By 1960 it had more than doubled, reaching 6.8 million. Today the population stands at 15.5 million. These figures are all the more remarkable when one learns that in 1938 the total number of doctors in British Government Service in Nigeria and the Gold Coast *combined* was 190. The Gold Coast had only eight African medical officers. In 1940 65,000 children attended schools in the Gold Coast, 2 per cent of the population. Albeit a small figure, it was far ahead of other West African states.[3] The pioneers of family planning in the yet-to-be-created nation of Ghana were among those children.

From June 1949 until Ghana's independence in March 1957, the nationalist struggle was led almost exclusively by the Convention People's Party (CPP) of Kwame Nkrumah who, as first leader of independent Ghana, was to impose his policies on the "society which was rooted in a traditional and extended pro-natalist family system".[4] Those who believed that both Ghana and Ghanaians would benefit from child spacing and planned families had to work quietly and slowly. The Christian Council of Ghana was the first group to initiate family planning information and services. Mrs Jean Forester-Payton, organized a medical advice centre for women which provided counselling and services in the early 1960s. The Ghana Midwives Association was another group which promoted family planning services early on. These and other groups later joined with doctors, social workers and well-known personalities to create the Planned Parenthood Association of Ghana (PPAG). Their motto: *Have Children by Choice, Not by Chance.* In 1966, this was a daring statement.

The story of family planning in Ghana is complex and rich with examples of individual commitment. It is a story of teamwork, timing and support from friends abroad. Because so many individuals were eager to support family planning work, a central co-ordinator was needed. Dr Barnor, the founder and President of the Ghana Medical Association, had experience in drawing people together for a common purpose. His willingness to act as the organizational back-up resulted in the creation of the PPAG. Dr Barnor's efforts went hand in hand with several associates among whom was Dr Augustus A. Armar who was later chosen to co-ordinate the government sponsored Ghana National Family Planning Programme (1970). Aided by countless friends and colleagues, the two doctors were among the principal architects of Ghana's current family planning programmes.

When I arrived to meet Dr M A Barnor, he was sitting in the patients' waiting room of the clinic he created in 1958. He led me to his office; before our meeting he had reviewed his records to look up the names of early collaborators. He admitted that this was the first time he had ever spoken of the strategy of creating the PPAG. Without knowing it, he was an able politician, who managed to involve key people in the cause of family planning before undertaking any initiatives. He owes his success perhaps to his soft-spoken manner and to the fact that he did not seek the limelight. Now in his mid-seventies, he still works each day in his hospital, the Link Road Clinic. Two of his five children are doctors; both daughters, they will one day take over his clinic. The sons, he said laughingly, were not interested in medicine.

Dr M. A. Barnor

"I grew up in Accra. I liked science and decided very early that I wanted to study medicine. I became a government scholar and was sent to Edinburgh University. Following studies there and at London University's School of Tropical Medicine, I returned to Ghana and entered the government medical service in 1949. Since I was a trained surgeon I was transferred every 18 months to different assignments. If you were a properly trained medical officer you could be posted to a remote place and be expected to do anything: obstructed labour, caesarean sections, fractures, intestinal obstructions. You had to know how to cope with everything – all sorts of emergencies.

"I was assigned to Accra, Kumasi, then was charged with reopening a hospital in Baquai. I was sent to the north, to Wa, where I had nearly one quarter the population of Ghana under my jurisdiction. You didn't have a chance to sit down; you had to go around to visit villages and do clinical work as well. So you were everything rolled into one. I ended up as Senior Medical Officer and hospital administrator in the Sekondi–Takoradi area in 1958. In between I went to Britain to do a post-graduate course. When I left government service in 1958, I had 10 years experience throughout the country. I set up this clinic and laboratory and I've been here ever since. Everybody thought I had arrived for the first time. They didn't know I knew Ghana because I had been to all the other regions; I had a good understanding of the medical situation of Ghana.

"I started a general practice here because there were very few practitioners around. In fact, the surroundings were just bush. The city has grown up around me. By the beginning of 1960 we were registering fifteen thousand new patients a year. There were many unwanted pregnancies and much illegal abortion. Women were having eight, 10, 12 pregnancies. They would come, tired, ill, not knowing there was an alternative. It was tragic. In Britain you could find contraceptives in chemists' shops. In Accra, here and there, you could find condoms discreetly sold. The chances of coming across oral tablets was remote. There was nothing organized and not even pharmacists were selling them. If they did, it was under the counter, because official policy was pro-natalist. The government wanted big families so birth control was virtually non-existent. Women came asking for advice. For most you had no answer. Some wanted abortions; others didn't ask for anything, they were just tired, weary of carrying pregnancies.

"It was due to this that family planning organizations started sending representatives to Ghana. The first representative I met was Edith Gates, who came here to this clinic in about 1959. Her trip was sponsored by the US-based Pathfinder Fund. She had begun coming here in 1956 and had spoken with many members of the medical establishment. She had tablets, foam rubber, various now-primitive things, of course. She talked about different family planning methods and about the desirability of initiating some kind of response to the problems we were facing. She was in touch with other people around the country but it didn't result in anything positive at that point: she was doing the ground work and when the situation would become propitious she would return.   She visited this clinic several times and left various contraceptive devices with me. By this time I think some pharmacists were beginning to stock oral contraceptives. But one did not know very much about it; so there was little knowledge or use of family planning.

"The person who really brought family planning concerns into prominence and consideration was Betty Hull. She was the IPPF Liaison Officer for Africa. She walked in one day without notice. I was then President of the Medical Association. She had worked for the University of Science and Technology in London and had been to Ghana before. She knew my brother, who was a registrar at the University. She was not, thus, a total stranger to Ghana. Her suggestions were welcome indeed; this would provide an answer for all the hapless women who were coming to see us and talk to us about their problems. She met with the Ministry of Health and the University of Ghana, people whom she considered would be interested in family planning. She found that civil servants, including doctors, showed interest but nothing concrete happened. In the face of official pro-natalist policy which wanted a remarkable jump in numbers, it was obviously risky in those days to undertake such a venture, and to risk being charged with 'ideological bankruptcy'. In those days and even now, family planning was regarded as a subtle device by the 'imperialists' to keep the country's population down.

"As President of the Ghana Medical Association I said I would attempt to sell the idea of child spacing in the context of Maternal and Child Health to the Association by stressing the risks of multiparity. It was hoped that medical men and women who believed in preventative medicine might be persuaded to form a family planning section within the Ghana Medical Association, as was allowed under the Constitution. We were both delighted that such a dodge had been found; it would allow family planning to be initiated by the Ghana Medical Association. It would thus have professional medical protection to withstand political storms that might arise as a consequence. Ms Hull mentioned the possibility of a family planning association but I didn't encourage her. I told her I didn't think it was a good idea given the stated policy was pro-natalist. That was January 1966.

"In February she left for the Ivory Coast. A few days later the Nkrumah government was overthrown by a *coup d'etat*. She wrote to me immediately. Had the situation changed enough to permit it? I replied I thought it had; the change in government made a tremendous difference. One was freer now, able to talk about family planning and invite people, to find out their views. The stage was set for the creation of an organization. We corresponded at length about how to start an association since we had agreed to move ahead into practicalities. She more or less led me through the practical steps to be taken.

"When I started in general practice, I spent my first ten years helping to build the Medical Association – perhaps I wasn't occupied enough, so I jumped into the creation of the PPAG.

Also, I had friends who were beginning to think in the same manner. It was important to make a conscious effort to talk to key people who might be interested – Dr. Bentsi-Enchill, Dr. Armar and others. Betty Hull had seen all of them, but they had not been in a position to do anything at the time. After hearing that I was in touch with a few sympathetic people, Ms Hull advised me about how to form an association, who to involve for specific reasons. We also needed somebody to go around and make the contacts with suitably interested persons. I chose Mrs. Konuah, an ex-pharmacist who was also a social worker. Her task was to identify the key people and I would tell her how to approach them. We were building a strategy.

"I contacted Dr Bentsi-Enchill. He said he would support me in anything I wanted to do – but as Head of the Department of Gynaecology, he was so busy he didn't have time to get actively involved. 'As long as I have your blessing,' I replied, 'I'm happy. If I call you to come to a meeting, just show yourself, that is all I need.' Dr Armar was in Kumasi. He, too, was sympathetic, very willing to get involved. In Accra we started with teachers at the Accra Academy. Little by little we brought in a group representing various professions. The midwives association was, of course, interested and became active participants. Soon we received an invitation from Ms Hull to attend the IPPF West European and Mediterranean Regional Conference in Copenhagen in July. Five Ghanaians were invited: two gynaecologists, Drs Bentsi-Enchill and Armar; a paediatrician, Dr Susan de Graft-Johnson, a General Practitioner, Dr M.A. Barnor and a Medical Statistician, Dr K.A. Saakwa Mante.

"The experience was eye-opening. Right then and there we decided that we would organize a family planning association as soon as we returned. Dr Armar wrote the report, which reads:

'The delegation came away from the Conference in Copenhagen in full agreement with objectives of the IPPF and determined to work towards bringing Ghana within the sphere of influence of that Federation by forming a National branch of the IPPF in the belief that through it, Ghanaians could be made to realize that:

1. Proper spacing of children is desirable so that parents may have children when they want them.
2. Too frequent child-bearing may injure maternal health and child development.
3. Improved health and nutrition of children can be achieved when mothers are free for as many years as they require to

nurture and feed their babies to promote healthy growth before the next baby arrives.

4. It is better for mothers to have 4 or 5 healthy live children properly looked after than 10, 11 or even 12 miserable children, 6 or more of whom may be lost through lack of proper care.

5. The incidence of criminal abortions could be significantly reduced if the incidence of unwanted pregnancies can be reduced by the judicious use of reliable contraceptives which can and should be made available to all mothers who may require them.

In our opinion there is a place for planned parenthood in Ghana.'

"The next step was to convene a meeting. It took place on August 27th. The convenors were Dr M.A. Barnor, Dr K.K. Bentsi-Enchill, Dr A.A. Armar, and Dr Susan de Graft-Johnson. The purpose was to create a country-wide planned parenthood organization. We had done the groundwork in the preceding months. It was clear that we should draft everyone that was interested into this movement. We invited our key target people some of whom subsequently became members of government. This helped bring government into the family planning concept. We opened branches, little by little with doctor friends. We did everything as it should be done. It was very efficiently run. There was no active opposition. We made it clear that we were not promoting a coercive programme. Socially I experienced comments, but not serious ones. Attitudes are still much the same although the younger generation is changing due to the economic situation. The unfortunate thing is that there are still some who are not convinced that family planning is a preventative, which leads to the reduction of abortions.

"On the government side, once the Nkrumah government's pro-natalist policy was scrapped there was nothing legal, for or against, family planning. The document which established the legality of family planning came later, in the 1969 two-year development plan where it was stated that government was going to support family planning services in conjunction with the Planned Parenthood Association of Ghana. The Department of Demography and Social Science had done some demographic surveys in the 1960s with funding from the Ford Foundation and the Population Council; they studied migration, mortality and fertility. Even in Nkrumah's time we had all the demographic data. In 1963, when they were writing the seven-year development plan, the planners told him that the facts showed that population growth would eliminate all economic growth if not controlled. They took a stand against the pro-natalist plan.

"Nkrumah appointed an inter-departmental committee in 1965 to study the question. This was about to be presented when his government was overthrown. When the military regime came into power 1967–69, they had all this information at their disposal. It facilitated their effort to come to the decision which brought forth the national population policy. The Health Chapter of the 1968 two-year development plan published stated: 'Government therefore, in co-operation with the PPAG, will provide family planning and fertility control services for those who desire them at all health facilities.' (page 94–95) The same year I was invited to sit on the Manpower Board, representing the PPAG. I declined and asked Fred Sai to go. He thus participated in the drafting of the official policy paper, namely, *Population Planning for National Progress and Prosperity* published in 1969. As a result of that, the National Family Planning Programme was inaugurated in 1969.

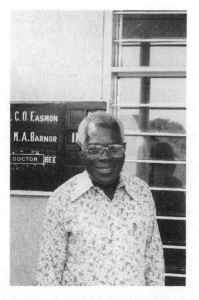

Dr M.A. Barnor standing before the Link Road clinic, Accra, Ghana, where he still practises medicine. Photographed by the author, January 1991.

"We had hospitals and health centres in operation with trained people in the Maternal and Child Health services. It was merely a question of asking these medical officers to add family planning to their work. Government wasn't going to have to establish new facilities. It was our intention right from the beginning that family planning services would be integrated with existing services. I must pay tribute to the government obstetricians for their early work. They co-operated with us; they were strong friends and we could rely on them. We owe so much to so many individuals who helped us along the way."

Dr Fred Sai

The current President of the International Planned Parenthood Federation (IPPF), Dr Fred Sai, was a member of the team of doctors and lay people who created the Planned Parenthood Association of Ghana (PPAG). Dr Sai's distinguished career as national and international civil servant culminated in his appointment to head the Office of Population at the World Bank, a post from which he retired in 1991.

"What is interesting about the start of family planning in Ghana is that unbeknown to each other a lot of people were, in fact, doing family planning for a long time. As the nutrition specialist of the country as of 1957, I had been working with my patients' mothers because I was seeing what was happening with marasmus or kwashiorkor cases. I was fitting diaphragms and advising on traditional contraceptives. I was also doing it for friends. But the government was against all this and one couldn't say anything to anybody. We Ghanaians had already realized that family planning was something that would be good for us. Among the doctors the motivation was the concern was for spacing births for maternal and child health. The patterns of weaning children were changing because of nuclearization of the family, urbanization, and that sort of thing. That, for me, was the number one concern. For the gynaecologists, it was the abortions they were seeing. Abortion, in my view, has always been a problem. It was not as extensive as it is now, but even when I was in secondary school, abortions were occurring. Few and far between but they were occurring. So abortion has always been there and with changes in social aspirations, the increase in the number of doctors and so on, abortions have become more frequent. This was a growing concern for gynaecologists.

"Others, like our demographer colleague Nelson Addo, were

seeing a more macro picture, the economic dimension of rapid population growth. We were thinking about all this but we had a government in power who was against family planning. We couldn't come out to form an association until that government changed. Everyone felt free again.

"At that time Ghanaians felt very strong in themselves. We were the first country to become independent; we had a good resource base, we had a good record. There was no reason why we wouldn't talk about these issues on an equal footing with others. People like Alan Guttmacher were moving around the world making statements on population and family planning. The Pathfinder Fund, from Clarence Gamble on, had been moving around. They weren't talking so much about a family planning association as much as family planning as a subject. The IPPF had decided as it were to proselytize a bit. It was sending consultants and staff out. So you had two efforts going on, one talking about family planning as such, and together trying to make people understand that a more formal structure would be a help.

"The volunteer tradition in Ghana is both external and internal. The chieftaincy system itself has a 'voluntary contribution' component that people have to make. You are allowed to work on your farm on so many days and on such and such day; if there is a road to be built, the chief will beat the gong and people will come and offer their services free. When the British raj was introduced, they tried to bring in the formalized sectors. For example, the secondary schools. Each school had a volunteer corps for going into villages to take care of nursing, or child care services, to demonstrate cropping patterns, that sort of thing. Then Girl Guides or Scouting were brought in, and the Red Cross came. Then, too, the Christian religion is something which encourages volunteer participation as well. All of these were planted on the fertile tradition of doing something communal for no pay. That tradition has been pretty strong.

"When we met to elect people to run the association, the doctors decided that this thing needed to be understood as a poor peoples' movement and not as a doctors' organization. The best way to assure that is to see that the top executives are lay people. The medical people can then be members of the committees and could chair the various sub-committees, the technical committees. I was given the Medical Committee. We gave the Education Committee to Susan de Graft-Johnson who was an obstetrician and was very concerned about all this. But since she was a Catholic, we didn't want to saddle her with anything which was more controversial than education. First she accepted but within a couple of months or so she gave her resignation, and some of us thought that you-know-who had talked to her."

Dr Augustus A. Armar

Obstetrician/gynaecologist, Dr Armar was affiliated to the Ghanaian Ministry of Health for fifteen years prior to being appointed to head the nationwide government initiative, the Ghana National Family Planning Programme. Dr Armar had been among those working quietly for a family planning programme, first a voluntary association and then the government initiative. He spent a year in the United States acquiring experience in family planning and fertility regulation, mainly at the Margaret Sanger Research Bureau in New York.

"I developed an interest in family planning originally due to the incidence of infertility and attempted abortions. As a gynaecologist and obstetrician I was sent to be at Kumasi. Home-made abortions were frequent. In many cases it consisted of drastic attempts to initiate the abortion process, to start the bleeding. Then the women could come to qualified medical personnel to complete the evacuation. Those who went to back street abortionists almost inevitably developed post-abortal pelvic infections due to lack of antibiotics. Since abortion was a very serious crime, we didn't see the cases until the women were in a very bad state. Terribly sad. Even on the verge of death, women would not reveal the identity of the person who had performed the abortion.

"As a gynaecologist obstetrician I had been doing family planning in the case of medical need for several years. When there was a clear medical indication that a woman would suffer severe health risks with another pregnancy, I would advise on contraception. I did it often on purely medical grounds. But I had come to the conclusion at that stage that there should be a fourth element in obstetric care: a family planning component. I don't think there is any self-respecting gynaecologist obstetrician who should discharge a patient from post-natal care without giving advice on family planning.

"Until 1966 you couldn't really talk about family planning in the open. You just dare not say anything about family planning for demographic reasons. The Nkrumah regime thought that more and more people were essential. But shortly after the *coup d'etat*, contacts became possible. Betty Hull returned to Ghana and got in touch with Dr Barnor and myself. I began to make contact with people abroad, with the Population Council, for example. Through them we made arrangements for the training of nurses for a post-partum programme family planning effort; these nurses eventually became the backbone of the country's family planning effort. Following the Copenhagen meeting, where we had been invited as a government delegation, I was charged with writing the report as the representative of the Health Ministry. Dr Barnor then organized a meeting here; I organized another in Kumasi and the PPAG was born.

"The government-sponsored effort, the Ghana National Family Planning Programme was conceived as one which would benefit by the incorporation of both government and private sector family planning initiatives. The Christian Council and the PPAG were in the private sector and the participating Ministries, like Health, Information and Education, were the government sector. The numerous agencies were each expected to contribute their own specific expertise to national goals. With all these agencies' participation, there was a need for co-ordination. The co-ordination function was assigned to the Secretariat of the National Family Planning Programme. That was what I was assigned to do."

Dr M A Barnor

1917   Born Accra, Ghana (Gold Coast)
1933-41 School at Mfantsipim and Achimota
1942-49 Edinburgh University and London School of Tropical Medicine
1949-58 Government Medical Service
1958   Opened private practice at Link Road Clinic
1959   Elected Honorary Secretary of Ghana Medical Association
1966   Appointed member of the National Liberation Council's Committee on Health
1967   Secretary–Convener of the Planned Parenthood Association of Ghana

References

1. J.F. Ade Ajayi and Michael Crowden, *History of West Africa*, Vol II
2. Sir Frederick Pedler, *Main Currents of West African History 1940-1978*, International College Editions, Macmillan, 1979
3. Ibid.
4. Planned Parenthood Association of Ghana, *1967-1977 10th Anniversary*, Chapter 2, Accra 1977

Chapter 12
Miyoshi Oba (b. 1921)

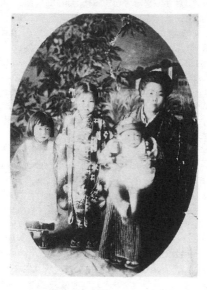

*Miyoshi Oba, second from left, with her mother and siblings,
Nagaro Province, Japan, circa 1927.*

The Iron-hearted lady

Miyoshi Oba won the affectionate name "iron-hearted lady"
when, at the age of 23 as the newly arrived public health nurse
in Takaho village, she dared address village women in a public
meeting. She had cast aside the tradition which permitted only
males to speak in public. But iron-hearted she was not. The
story of her accomplishments during a 35-year career as a public health nurse is proof of the kindness and caring she gave to
all. On a recent visit to Takaho village, Susaka City and Nagano,
I saw with what admiration and affection she is surrounded.

The year before Miyoshi Oba was born, Shidzue Kato, one
of the founders of modern family planning, was already working with Margaret Sanger to broaden the international family

planning movement. Renowned worldwide for her devotion to the cause of women's health and well-being through family planning, Kato, now 92, is President of the Family Planning Association of Japan and recipient of the highest distinctions for international family planning work. Miyoshi Oba is of those who followed the courageous example of Shidzue Kato. As a young public health nurse Miyoshi Oba was assigned to one of the poorest villages in Japan, Takaho. It was 1943. The village was plagued with poverty and poor health. Notions of hygiene were rudimentary; tuberculosis, parasites and communicable diseases were common. So were abortions.

Before and during World War II, the Japanese were urged to have as many children as possible. To advocate the use of contraceptives was to risk jail. Five to six children per family was the norm.[1] At the end of the war, poor food distribution coupled with raging inflation left people malnourished; infant mortality stood at 76.7 per 1000.[2] In 1950 the government, which feared a rapid increase of Japan's population, changed the law and abortion became legal. Sadly, contraception remained unknown and unavailable in most areas of the country. By 1952 there were two and a half times as many abortions as live births. In the prefecture where Ms Oba worked, it was found that 39 women had three or more abortions in 1950 alone.[3] Ms Oba, as a young unmarried nurse who had never seen or heard of a condom, decided something had to be done to reduce the reliance on abortion. She was to spearhead a family planning campaign by providing both information and contraceptives. Organizational abilities, coupled with her sensitivity to traditions, proved invaluable in creating the climate and structures to provide the villagers of Takaho with the knowledge and means to improve health and plan their families. She created a network of health workers, trained other nurses, introduced notions of hygiene, nutrition, public health and family planning to villagers who had hitherto been ignorant of basic health care.

These conversations took place in the spring of 1991. We wish to thank Ms Aiko Iijima of the Japanese Organization for International Co-operation in Family Planning, Inc. for her assistance in serving as interpreter.

Miyoshi Oba

"I was born on the 'Day of Ebisu God'. He is famous for his happy face and smile. So my mother used to say to me, 'You should always be happy with a smile on your face'. It was the

Taisho era, 1922. My mother was 20 years older than me. She got married at the age of 19 and gave birth to her first baby the next year. She bore eight children in all. Since I was the first child my mother always said to me, 'If you are a good child, all the others will become good. Since you are the eldest, you have to set an example for your younger brothers and sisters. You have to look after the younger ones. When you answer, you have to pronounce 'Yes' very clearly. Don't repeat it like 'Yes, yes' only one 'Yes' is good. You have to say 'Itadakimasu' when you eat, and 'Gochiso-sama' [words expressing gratitude] when you finish. So, in the morning if you say 'Ohayo' [good morning], the others will also say 'Ohayo'. If you do such things, the younger ones will follow.' My parents said if I did not observe this discipline, I would not be able to cope with people in society.

"Another good thing I remember about my parents was that they always gave the same things we ate to poor people who came begging for food or drink. They said that everyone becomes hungry and thirsty like us. When poor people came, they invited them inside the house and treated them like family members. Sometimes as children, we were disappointed to see nothing left from what we had kept for our after-school snack. When we asked about it, my mother would say 'Today so-and-so came with an empty stomach, so I gave it to them. If you do a good thing, people will help you when you are in trouble.' But if we did something wrong, father'd smack us.

"It sounds strange now, but in those days no girls in rural areas went to senior high school. The highest level of education was two years after primary school (six years in all). Most girls discontinued their formal education after primary school and began to work. Although my family was poor, my father readily bought books for me. There was not much reading material in those days, except monthly magazines for girls, such as *Girls' Club*. So I got a subscription and seriously perused them. Seeing me reading all the time, my parents were happy to buy books for me. My father told me to study further so that I could obtain professional skills and become 'independent'. He said, 'From now on even a woman should be able to stand on her own feet, otherwise she may be faced with miserable situations. So if you want to obtain some professional skills we will support you even if we encounter difficulties.' He suggested two options: to study two years after primary school and enter a teacher's college, or to train as a midwife.

"I decided to become a midwife. I wanted to become independent and to earn money as soon as possible to support the younger brothers. I might have been influenced to opt for the health-related line of midwife because of my father's experience in pharmaceutical work. I don't know, but I do know it was too ambitious for me to become a doctor. The fees for training professionals were not very expensive. But nobody in the rural area could afford university tuition. My father had wanted to study himself, but because his family was very poor, he could not get the higher education he had wished for. To me he said, 'If you do not have the ability to continue, I don't mind if you abandon your studies; but if you are capable enough, and wish to do so, I will use all my efforts and sacrifice whatever is needed.'

"My father was a farmer initially. But he was a farsighted person and wanted to do something else. Eventually he started a pharmacy with his younger brother. It cost a fortune to do it. He invested all the money from the sale of his farming land in it. But too young and inexperienced, the brothers did not succeed in the business. My father gave the shop to his younger brother and my parents went to work in a coal mining area. Because of that, I had some difficult times in my childhood. I had to live with my grandparents and with three younger siblings for about five years. I was eight years old. My grandparents took care of us until I finished primary school.

"When I finished senior primary school (the two years following primary school) I stayed at home for two years, as I thought it necessary to help my grandmother with chores. During the two years at home I sometimes attended the youth class. But I was not satisfied, and my father thought it better for me to have the formal education sooner because he knew I was very eager to continue studying. In Nagano City the Shinano Health Association (equivalent to the present Department of Health) used to conduct a one-year training course for nurses and midwives. So I took the examination for the training course and passed it. After completing the course, trainees could become either a nurse or midwife, provided that she passed the qualifying examination. I passed them both. I wanted to attend the Nurses College associated with Tokyo University but I would have to work for one year in Tokyo to earn the tuition. My parents agreed with the idea, if it was my wish. I asked a friend to find a hospital near Tokyo University. She introduced me to the chief nurse of Jippi clinic and I began work there.

"When I finished training as a public health nurse, I was assigned to work at the Kanda Public Health Centre. But it was wartime and my family was worried about my safety. As

I was the eldest child, my family told me to come home even for a short time, until the end of the war. You know everybody believed Japan would win the war. I went back home, expecting that it would be only for a short time, until the war ended in victory. So on 31 March 1943 as a public health nurse [PHN] I went home to Nagano Prefecture, as my family had urged me to do.

"Public health nurses had begun to be highly regarded and were assigned at the village level. From Tokyo I was assigned to the Nagano City Public Health Center. But it took a whole day commuting between my house in Nire village and the health centre in Nagano. It was already noon by the time I arrived at the centre. It was then that a post came available at the next village, Takaho village; the village head was a remote relative. I began work there right away. The village was very poor. There were no health services. It was just like the situation in developing countries such as Vietnam now, because Japan was in the middle of the war at that time. I was the first public health nurse in Takaho village. People did not know what to call a public health nurse. Some called me the 'health woman'. They knew about midwives or traditional birth attendants, but they did not know what to expect from a public health nurse.

"I was 22 years old. I wanted to do so much. I was full of hope for the future. I wanted to bring infant mortality down to zero. I was idealistic and tried to work for future goals. I thought Japan would win the war and I expected to go back to Tokyo when the war was over. I wanted to do everything quickly so that it would be done by the time I left the village for Tokyo. The villagers used to say, 'You are always so busy, rushing about. You don't take enough time to bow your head lower, to make polite greetings.'

"There were no doctors. Actually, there was one doctor but he was crippled. There were no telephones except one in the village office. Many babies died because of diarrhoea. People used to drink from the river. There were parasitic infections and many communicable diseases. I thought it should be me who changed the villagers' lives for the better.

"Although I myself had led the same kind of life there before, I realized that much change and improvement was necessary. I wanted to prevent communicable diseases, to improve nutrition, and even though there was hardly anything to eat, to help plan nutritious crops. And I wanted to educate young people because they would be the ones to carry on the new ideas. The villagers expected me to be able to do everything: immunization, injections, midwifery and so on. As someone who had been trained in Tokyo, I was supposed to be able to do many things quickly, respond to the people's requests skillfully and efficiently and visit the people in need immediately. People's awareness of health issues was low so I had to start with good health education. They needed to change their daily habits if health were to be improved, but how to approach this issue was the problem. I decided to ask if the women's group would let me speak at their meetings, because I had been taught this as a strategy in school.

"It was totally unusual for a woman to speak in public. For example, if the Chairperson of the Women's Association organized a group meeting and invited the mayor as a speaker, she sat next to the speaker and sometimes bowed silently. That was all. Later the mayor told me that he had been worried about what I was going to do when I asked him to take me to a women's gathering to speak about health education. I spoke about nutrition and then asked the women in audience, 'Those who eat dried fish please raise your hand'. I wanted to explain that dried fish is good for calcium. Only one person, a midwife, raised her hand. I learned a big lesson that day. I felt very shameful when I realized the people were so poor they could not afford to buy dried fish. With all the knowledge that I learned at school, I couldn't improve health conditions in the community without knowing the reality of people's lives. It was useless to dump school teachings on village people. The important thing is to understand people's thinking quickly and then find ways to meet their true needs, to know how to get others' assistance for that purpose, how to get co-operation from others. Alone, a PHN cannot do much. She should work behind the scenes. She should not be the only actor on the stage. People themselves should be the main actors.

"Without knowing how to mobilize others, no good work can be done. This is the principle of promoting public health. It is natural that everyone likes to get attention from others when some good work is done. So it is important to give recognition in public that thanks to *this* and *that* person – even if you, the PHN, made the most efforts. In this way, people are happy. Since an honorable occasion does not happen often in peoples' lives, they will always remember the event happily. Isn't that much better than only one person being the creator of everything? I think my mother tried to teach me that principle, but I was not serious enough to understand the true meaning of what she said in those days.

"My mother was an ordinary woman, but when she died more

than five hundred people came to the funeral ceremony. I was surprised. She was an ordinary mother in a rural area but many people came to say that they had much to be thankful to her for. She didn't have a higher education. She came from a family which for generations had been doctors from the domain of Matsushiro, in the Nagano area, where Sanada was the feudal lord. She often said, 'Your ancestors were doctors and used to help people, and so it is good that you are also helping the people. If you do so you, too, will be helped by others.'

"One day I was asked by the prefectural government to accept a position at the Prefectural Health Department. I immediately consulted the head of the village, saying, 'I don't know what to do, because I don't want to leave the village'. He asked, 'Are you sure that you don't want to accept the offer? Do you really want to stay in the village and continue to work here?' I said, 'Yes, I want to stay here.' 'If so,' he replied, 'please do stay and share the task of improving poor conditions here. It is a very hard task, as you know. If you go to the prefectural office, you can get a better salary with better working conditions. But if you prefer to continue to work here, then please stay with us. It is a very difficult job but I will do my best to support you.' I was so moved with these words that I made my decision on the spot and conveyed my answer to the prefectural government.

"During the war, there were no doctors in Takaho village. Villagers would come to see me at the village office when someone was ill. I would then telephone the doctor who lived outside the village. When he arrived with his car, I took him to all the homes of the sick. It was usually midnight before I returned home. I didn't mind such hard work because I believed it was my duty. I was young and healthy.

"During the war there were no men in the village, so women had to do everything. But even before the war, conditions were not better. The village was said to be one of the poorest villages in the country, because the silk industry in which the villagers were engaged had declined. The women's work was very hard. They worked from early morning till late at night. Women were anaemic, exhausted, had stiff shoulders, and very scarce breast milk. They couldn't eat enough fish because food was on short rations.

"Many people came to see me complaining about abdominal pain. I myself had many worms, too. People utilized human manure that was not yet rid of parasites for fertilizer at that time. Almost 100 per cent of the people were infected with parasites. People also used the stagnant water of the river for their daily life. There were many fleas and lice, and people could not sleep well at night. So those who were able to survive must have been very strong.

"I consider myself fortunate to have been able to help people with parasite control under those conditions because my relationship with the people was made very close. This experience has been utilized in other Asian and developing countries, utilizing parasite control as the entry point of family planning and maternal and child health and of increasing the good relations between the health workers and the people.

"There were many couples who had a dozen children, but usually two or three children died of diarrhoea, pneumonia or infectious diseases. And there were many problems between men and women. They did not mix in those days. Most marriages were arranged. A proper bride and bridegroom did not look at each other. There were cases where a couple saw each other's face only the morning after their marriage ceremony. Before the war, Japan was a feudalistic society. Since the war things have slowly changed for the better. A lot of these pregnancies were not wanted after the war. Before the war national policy was to have many children. After the war, however, democracy was applied to Japan, thanks to the policy of the American Occupation Forces. Many nurses came to Japan from the United States to give guidance about various matters such as family planning, maternal health, and initiation of Mother's Clubs. We were taught how we should promote our work in a democratic way. Eventually people in the village began to realize how important it was for them to provide their children with education.

"So many things began to change after the war ended in August 1945. It was also after the war that public health centres were built and a health promotion system was established. In 1948 the Eugenic Protection Law was established. Under this law one could get an abortion easily; many people began to rely on abortion. Before the war even if the women's health was poor it was impossible to get abortion. Furthermore, although they did not like to become pregnant, they did not know how to practise family planning. There were many self-induced abortions. It was said, for example, that drinking furnace ashes boiled in water was effective for abortion. Others inserted a stick into their vagina. But generally people strongly believed that children were a treasure for parents, and that if a pregnancy occurred it was very natural for the woman to give birth to the baby. If some artificial intervention was made, it was considered sinful.

At night parents and children slept in the same room. Men were always dominant. Men drank a lot, and were not co-operative in practising family planning. It did not work well at times in the village. Men and women were not at all equal; I think women sacrificed a lot. That is why I decided to form the Mandarin Duck Club (Mandarin Ducks are famous and admired because once they choose a mate they always stay together) inviting both husband and wife. It was no use if only victims gathered and discussed their problems, although they used to gather together and grumble about men. It was more important to get the wrongdoers together as well.

"It was difficult to involve men in the club; I had to think strategically. I decided the most important thing was to get support from the village head and other village leaders such as the Chief of Agricultural Co-operatives, and the Chief of the Fire Brigade. I approached the village headman first. I wanted the village administration to promote the idea because it was a village problem. I told the leaders that we had to do something to improve the situation. Otherwise wives would die and many men would become widowers. At the time the number of abortions was higher than that of live births.

"I tried to mobilize all resourceful persons, and finally it was approved. They were very supportive of my idea of involving men in family planning, as pregnancy is not caused only by women. I involved the Agricultural Co-operatives; they were strong economically and I expected them to help with contraceptives supplies later. I approached the Chief. There was also a very good doctor whose mind was very broad. He was very humorous and good at persuading the others on private matters such as family planning. He was very supportive of my idea.

"You know I saw a condom for the first time in my life when I attended a family planning study meeting. Isn't it funny that such a person was promoting family planning? I was not married, so I could not talk about how people felt about using condoms. I asked Dr Matsuzawa to talk about it. He was very good at talking about such subjects. He said that if one wears a condom it is like when one takes a hot spring bath putting boots on the feet, or something like shaking hands with gloves on. Given this, I thought that the best thing was to find out how to use the least number of condoms, that is, to use condoms only during the time in the menstrual cycle when a woman was most likely to get pregnant. So I thought of having study meetings to learn what should be the shortest period that the couple had to use contraceptives. With this purpose I would be able to motivate people to come to study meetings.

"I asked Dr Takano from the Health Department of Nagano Prefecture to speak about condoms at the Mandarin Club. He said that wearing condoms one could get excitement, and a climax could be reached. It was a matter of technique. 'And' he said, 'If it takes a little longer you can enjoy sex more.' Some people believed that if women didn't get any semen in them, they would not get the hormone and it would make them frigid. Or if the husband took a long time to have a climax, the wife would become impatient. Since such questions were the subject of medical science, I asked Dr Ishigaki, who is a famous doctor, to answer them when he was invited as a guest speaker. He explained that hormones are transfused through blood, not from something expelled outside the body.

"I promoted the idea that women should help men put on the condom. While the penis was big enough, they should remove it. These things are to be done by women with love and tender care. They must be thankful because, if not, if a man doesn't use a condom, it's women who suffer. The men and women of the Mandarin Duck Club discussed these things together in a very friendly and democratic way. Usually some member started mentioning his or her case and others reacted, discussed it and reached a conclusion. For example, someone asked what is the best way to wear a condom? Then another answered, 'You know, in my case, my wife puts the condom on me.' Then the others said, 'That's a very good idea. Let's try that.' Some of them were very frank in telling about their private life.

"So all decisions were made by the couples. I tried to give them useful knowledge and information, but the decisions came out of the group. We had a very good leader, named Dr Matsuzawa. He knew what needed to be done and persuaded people in a nice manner and with a lot of humour.

"We organized exchanges in family planning promotion within the prefecture. We sent our couples [Mandarin Duck Club members] to speak on the importance of the involvement of husband and wife in family planning promotion so that others would follow that idea. The husbands' understanding towards their wives began to increase. One day, as a thank you to their wives, they decided to cook for their wives at a meeting.

"You know men are very shy and they used to come to the meetings with a bit of alcohol and in a happy mood. Sometimes they decided some extraordinary thing and then afterwards were surprised to learn what they had decided. But generally the meeting was conducted under a very happy and friendly atmosphere. They also tested condoms during the meetings. They tried to use cigarette smoke and test the condoms together with their wife, saying to the wife, 'Look, isn't it all right? there is no hole!' Condoms were always a big issue for discussion. For instance, many condoms were found floating in the creek. We discussed where to dispose of them and where to keep them. In order to dispose of the condoms, it was suggested that it be wrapped in a sheet of newspaper and burned. They discussed how to have a sex life without being disturbed by children, while sleeping all in one room. One said, 'We usually hit the children on their head one by one, to make sure they are sound asleep.'

"Condoms were in great demand. They were sold through a unique system of passing a small box, called a 'love box' from house to house. A love box contained condoms but appeared to be an ordinary medicine chest. It was disguised to fool the children. Ten to fifteen households shared a love box, which was circulated according to the order of the names. When the box is delivered, the person takes out as many condoms as required, puts the money for them into a small slot in the box and sends it on to the next person on the list. If the box is empty, they apply for a new supply from the public health nurse at the village office. One day when such supplies were collected by a husband and were being carried by bicycle, they were dropped in the street and I got a report from the police for that.

"Today, the public health nurses of Suzaka City sit in the front offices. Before we were placed behind other staff. Since we fought against other administrative officials to solve difficult problems that faced people, the officials put us behind them so that such matters were not disclosed to the public. I went to see the mayor and said, 'Sir, you are the leader of this village and the most powerful person here, but you are still not be able to enter the bedrooms of the villagers. We, the public health nurses, can enter their bedroom to protect their health. So you should put us nearest to the people in the office.' He immediately agreed with me.

"What makes me happy is to hear that the young public health nurses of the villages are doing a fine job. Then I feel that I have done something good for the people."

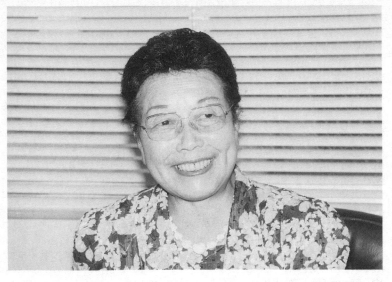

*Miyoshi Oba, retired Public Health Nurse and promoter of
planned parenthood since the 1940s, pictured here in 1991.*

Group discussion 20 May 1991 in Suzaka City, Nagano Prefecture

The following comments were made during a luncheon honoring
Ms Oba at the Susaka City offices of the Nagano Prefecture.
Half a dozen former colleagues of Ms Oba joined in to comment
on her style and work.

Mr Yamashita was Head of the Health Division from 1969
to 1981 for 12 years: "In the beginning I did not know much
about health, but gradually I learned from Ms Oba about
the importance of health. It was the same with our mayor.
He used to cut our health budget but gradually he began to
approve what we proposed. In other words, Ms Oba trained us
to become aware of the importance of the health programme."

Mrs Kobayashi is a public health nurse who worked with Ms
Oba: "Ms Oba was very good at encouraging and motivating
other people to work. Suzaka City was famous for its active
public health nurses. She was about 46 years old at the time
I arrived here. She was excellent at promoting team work. She
never ordered us to do things. She let us think and take action
on our own, so we could always work with a happy feeling.

"As for talking about family planning, she was very good, very straightforward. I learned that if the speaker shows some hesitation or some feelings of embarrassment in talking about family planning, the audience, too, becomes embarrassed. But if we speak very frankly and openheartedly, people feel more comfortable and become open with the issue."

Mrs Uehara is a former member of Health Promoters' Association: "Ms Oba did not use the word 'condom' but 'Furisode', the name for a beautiful kimono with long sleeves that young girls wear on special happy occasions such as a wedding ceremony or graduation ceremony. Another nickname for the condom was 'iris'. So when I became a member of the Health Promoters' Association, I thought that the members should distribute the seeds of the flower among the people. When I asked her about it, she said to me, "No, you see, you are not distributing the seeds but the bags in which to put the seeds."

Miyoshi Oba

1921	Born Nagano Prefecture, Japan
1939	Graduated from Nurse and Midwifery Training
1945	Stationed as Public Health Nurse in Takaho Village
1952	Participated in Training Course for Family Planning Promoters and becomes qualified family planning worker
1982	After retirement, works as part-time public health nurse at Suzaka City
1951–90	Received number of awards for public health work

References

1&3. JOICFP, *Where There is a Will*, the story of a Countryside Health Nurse, JOICFP Document Series 3, 1981.
2. Ministry of Health and Welfare, *Statistics relating to Maternal and Child Health in Japan*, 1988.

Chapter 13
Dr Faran Samaké
(1932 – 1978)

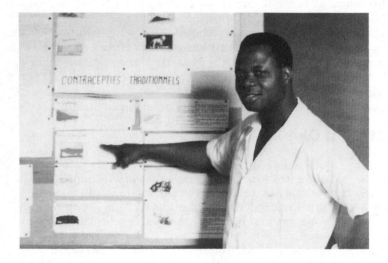

Dr Faran Samaké, a pioneer of family planning in Mali, teaching a course in reproductive health in Bamako, 1962.

Everyone knew that if they had a problem, someone would say, 'Go see Dr Faran.' This is how he came to be concerned about family planning.
Mme Sokona Diabaté

Mali is a land-locked nation astride the southern Sahara desert and the African Sahel; poor in natural resources and subject to cyclical drought, it is a nation of herders and small farmers. It is a land of learned tradition going back to the Mandingo Empire, which flourished in the 13th–15th centuries. From the early Middle Ages, caravans crossed the desert headed for trading posts in North Africa and Arabia. Due to the strong Arab influence, a large portion of Mali's people are Muslims. In the late nineteenth century the French built a fort at Bamako, the present-day capital, and in 1893, Mali was made part of the French Sudan, the culmination of French domination of what was then known as French West Africa. When Mali became an autonomous state in 1958, its population stood at a little over three million people. Today, of the nine million Malians, 46 per cent are under 14 years of age.

The drought of 1984–85 had devastating consequences for Mali. Millet, sorghum and maize production declined by more than 50 per cent and hundreds of thousands of people left their homes in search of food. The nomadic population, which lives primarily on raising livestock lost 40 and 80 per cent of their animals. Mali relies on the export of cotton and livestock to earn foreign exchange but even in a good year, the value of exports earns about half of required imports. With a foreign debt of $1,847 million and a per capita income of $270, Mali faces a precarious future.

In 1972, Mali became the first francophone West African nation to repeal the 1920 French law restricting the right to contraceptive use. The account of how the law was repealed and of how family planning was made available in Mali is one of teamwork. A young psychiatrist, Dr Faran Samaké, was the team leader. All those who speak of Dr Samaké's achievements refer to his ability to persuade others to collaborate. When the young doctor returned to Mali following studies in France, he, like many of his colleagues, found the French colonial legacy too restrictive; the law banned the promotion and use of contraceptives. Knowing that he would be unable to challenge the legal code by himself, Faran Samaké convinced others to join him. The effort was to take over five years. With the support of two key colleagues, Sidi Coulibaly, an economist, and Ina Sissoko, an official in the Ministry of Social Affairs, the law was finally changed. Family planning was legalized and the way was cleared for the creation of Association Malienne pour la Promotion et la Protection de la Famille (AMPPF). Mme Sy, the chief midwife of Bamako's maternity hospital, was another member of the team. She organized early support of midwives whose endorsement of family planning gave confidence to the women of Mali.

Dr Samaké died suddenly in 1978 at the age of 46. Those quoted here tell the story of a remarkable man who is considered the pioneer of many medical advances in Mali.

Sidi Coulibaly, an economist, is retired from government service. I met him at his home early one December morning in

1990. With him was his neighbour and former colleague, Abdou Tourkara, a statistician who recently retired as Head of Programmes at the AMPPF.

Sidi Coulibaly

"I started working with Dr Samaké in 1967 but I was interested in family planning long before that. There was an active movement for the legalization of family planning in France, when I was a student there from 1959 to 1966. Both contraception and abortion were illegal, so those who had money travelled either to England or Switzerland for abortions. For others, the poor, there was no help. They resorted to abortions in very dangerous conditions.

"I was particularly influenced by a near tragedy I witnessed. A very close friend had gone to Mali on vacation and had sexual relations with his fiancée. She became pregnant. They were terrified by this 'accident' since in our society, it meant a major scandal. My friend paid the girl's way to Paris and, then, to assure secrecy of the abortion, it was performed in my room at the Cité Universitaire. She haemorrhaged badly. Luckily, because there were many medical students living in the dormitory, she was saved. But it might well have been a tragedy. This, to me, was a cruel form of social injustice. The laws forbidding contraceptives were based on moral and religious hypocrisy. The next day I went out and joined the French family planning movement. I went to all sorts of meetings and demonstrations to get family planning legalized. I had a membership card from the students' movement for family planning.

"When I returned to Mali in 1966, Dr Faran Samaké got in touch with me. We had known each other years before. He was the kind of fellow who was always joking, always in a good mood. If you met him you would think he didn't take anything seriously but in reality, when Faran had an idea in his head, he usually got his way. The idea this time, was the legalization of family planning. He was then chief of the psychiatric ward at Point-G Hospital. He was also responsible for health in the prison system. In both the prisons and the psychiatric institutions, men and women are poorly separated. There were a great many unwanted pregnancies. This created a moral dilemma for Dr Samaké because, in some cases, it was necessary to perform abortions. This may very well be the origin of his interest in family planning.

"Knowing of my interest, he contacted me and said, 'We

are going to create a family planning association and we will need an economist, a demographer, sociologist, etc.' He had constituted a group of like-minded individuals through personal contacts. We were all different. Some were interested in family planning for health reasons, others on humanitarian grounds and still others, economists like myself, who foresaw the consequences of demographic trends on the development of our country. Remember, if in 1966 you suggested that there might be a demographic problem in Mali, people couldn't understand. They would reply, 'Mali has 1,200,000 km^2 of land; it can hold lots more people'. They forget that half of Mali is desert, that it is more the rate of growth than the number of inhabitants per square kilometre that is at issue. The higher the population growth rate, the more capital you have to invest if you want to improve the standard of living for that population. I could see that with Mali's population growth rate and the investments we would be able to make, the standard of living could only get worse. This was not easily understood at the time – and it remains unaccepted or misunderstood by many even today. That was the second reason for my militantism for family planning.

"So, as a friend of Faran Samaké, I agreed to become involved in his two-pronged strategy. The first activity was to create a family planning association and we succeeded fairly quickly. Then we were to lobby for the legalization of family planning. Once that was accomplished, the President of the Republic, Mr Traoré, understood our objectives and gave us his support. Our second concern was education. Everything from neighbourhood meetings to, later on, use of the radio. We tried to make ourselves known to the greatest number of people as we expanded our services.

"Dr Faran Samaké was an amazingly energetic and sociable man. Because of his profession and his outgoing personality, he knew people in all walks of life, in all levels of society. And he didn't pay much attention to hierarchy. When the Minister of Health didn't want to help create the association, Faran went around him to the Minister of Social Affairs, Ina Sissoko. As soon as we got a green light from her, we went ahead. She helped us with our campaign and arranged for us to participate in training workshops abroad.

"We learned from others' experience what to do and what not to do in setting up a family planning association: how did others' initiate their programmes, how were they accepted by the public, what should we avoid doing so as not to alienate or shock public opinion. What support should we seek. We needed doctors and medical personnel, opinion leaders such as religious and political figures. But first, we had to change the law banning contraceptives. On the 28th of June 1971 the French law which forbade family planning was abolished. The Association could exist legally and provide contraceptive services.

"We had learned from others that you can't motivate people unless you offer good services at the same time. We began thus by opening a pilot family planning centre. The consultations there were not limited to contraceptive services; all women's health problems were treated. We had medicines for a whole range of illnesses. We wanted to demonstrate that family planning is a part of general health care. We took all sorts of legal precautions in setting up the association: we stated, for example, that women needed the authorization of their husband in order to benefit from our contraceptive services. For unmarried girls, parental authorization was required. This is true even today. But the precautions did not eliminate opposition or misunderstanding.

"At the outset we had some opposition from women. A delegation went to see the President of the Republic to denounce the creation of the AMPPF, which had been legally founded and accepted by the government. The President explained that there was no reason to oppose such an association, since family planning is voluntary. Men, also, were opposed. They believed that access to contraceptives would encourage prostitution and extramarital relations. This warranted a huge educational effort which continues even now. One of the principal barriers to family planning was the belief that a multitude of children is equated with abundance and prosperity. When infant mortality was very high, people had large families as insurance against child death. That, and the religious belief that children are a gift from God and that God doesn't give you children that you can't care for, were the two major factors for having large families. Even if they saw their children die of hunger, the belief remained strong in the minds of most Malians. Now, with the difficult economic situation, that is changing.

"Despite these objections – which still exist – family planning is fully integrated in the Maternal and Child Health programmes of the Ministry of Health. I worry now because we are witnessing an increase in the influence of conservative religious teachings, in fundamentalism. This could jeopardize the family planning effort because political leaders seem to base their attitude to family planning on what they believe to be public opinion. It happened to me in the beginning. When I came back to Mali. A friend said, 'Sidi, if you want to run for office, be part of the political party, you won't have a chance if you get involved in family planning'. He was wrong. Those who were courageous enough to go ahead were able to convince the government, and family planning is now accepted by the great majority of the people.

"Today, theoretically, the government has a population policy but in practice, it doesn't dare undertake a true population policy. It doesn't clearly say to Malians, 'Look, the population growth rate is too high for the quantity of fertile land we possess. We are moving towards catastrophe."

Ina Sissoko

Mme Sissoko is currently a Technical Adviser to the Ministry of Employment in Bamako. As I sat interviewing her in her office, anyone who put their head through the door was greeted with jokes and friendly teasing. A member of Dr Faran Samaké's team, she recalled her involvement in the legalization of family planning when, as the Minister for Social Affairs, she introduced the required statutes.

"The moral distress of women I witnessed as Minister of Social Affairs affected me deeply. My commitment came from seeing their plight. I had set up a system whereby from 3 pm on every Friday, I received visits from anyone who needed to talk with an official of the Social Affairs Ministry. Sometimes alone, sometimes in groups, women would come to see me, with their problems. One of those women, in particular, made me realize the human tragedy of unwanted pregnancies. She sat in front of my desk holding a child which was nursing at her breast. She was 38 years old and illiterate. She looked at me with great sad eyes and said, 'Madame how I wish I wouldn't have any more children. My husband is a drunkard. When he gets paid he gives me a little and then disappears until he has spent all the rest. Then he comes back to me. I try to raise my children as best I can in these conditions but I have eight. Eight of them! – I don't know how I can go on. My husband is always drunk; I have to fend for the children by myself, feed them, teach them. I don't want any more. I can't go on.' Seeing her, drained of her health and hope, I decided to try to do something about family planning in Mali. Contraceptives existed but they were only available through private doctors and they cost a great deal. No poor woman could ever afford them.

"Faran Samaké used to come to my office and we'd discuss all sorts of things. His social conscience was practically visible, it was so strong. When he said he wanted to start a family planning association, I said 'Go ahead, I'll back you'. I could help him with the idea and from within the government but he was the one who really started the association, who got everything going.

"About that time, a Canadian gentleman, M. Le Plante, was making the rounds of the different ministries so I told him of our plans to start an association. He said that the Canadian International Development Agency (CIDA) could help out by inviting interested Malians to Canada to see how they had started their family planning programme. He arranged for four Malians to go to Canada for a training session: Coulibaly, Faran Samaké were among them. When they returned we agreed that the first thing to do was to change the law to permit legalized family planning. With the help of several colleagues, I formulated a policy document which provided the legal framework for family planning and government policy.

"I was the only woman in the 15-member Council of Ministers. The proposed legislation had been distributed well before the meeting so that everyone had time to study it. Of course, I was the one to present it. Only two members present were willing to support me: Mr Coulibaly and the former director of Mali's Development Bank. When I finished my presentation, the President opened the discussion. Arguments ranged from 'Mali is a very large country and is in need of people to work and develop the economy.' Others were worried about the 'cost of a family planning policy'. The Minister of Health said his Ministry had not been consulted. If they had been, he stated, 'We, the doctors, would have objected to family planning as a government policy. It is a dangerous policy for Mali. Dangerous from a financial, moral and religious point of view. It is against Islamic principles.'

"We responded 'Wait a minute, Tunisia and Egypt have family planning programmes and they are Muslim countries.' Then we pointed out that family planning also intended to help women who wanted children and faced infertility problems. The President let everyone speak and then said, 'I think we should accept the proposal presented by Mme Sissoko. A need exists; it is a social reality which we must confront. We must have children who are strong and well-educated, who can help the development of Mali. I promised Mme Sissoko that this law would be passed so that family planning is available in Mali. I keep my promises.'

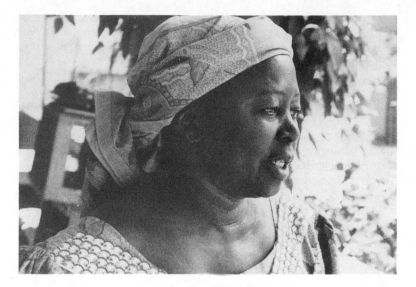

Ina Sissoko, Technical Adviser to the Ministry of Employment (Mali) and a pioneer in family planning, talking with the author in Bamako, 1990.

"That is how the law was adopted. It was by authority of the President, for most of the others were against it. Those were difficult times for all of us but we won the day. I worked from within the administration, as did Coulibaly. Faran prodded from outside. Without him we couldn't have garnered the support. He was such a generous man. People came to Bamako from his region and he would never refuse them. I'd see him go by in the morning on his way to the hospital; his car full of patients. His death was a great loss for Mali."

Sokona Diabaté Sy

Mme Sy is without a doubt the most famous midwife of Mali. As chief midwife of the maternity hospital in Bamako and one of the first volunteers of the Malian family planning association, she was a member of Dr Faran's team. She is now retired, although still active as a volunteer in the family planning association. We met at her home in the early evening. As we sat in her sitting room, drinking pineapple soda she reminisced about events 20 years ago.

"Dr Faran was a wonderful doctor. He loved people and was so kind-hearted that everyone went to him. Many women went to him for abortions. Fathers, mothers, young girls – all could go to him to seek counsel and help.

"In the early 1970s all of us agreed that we needed a family planning programme. We were both members of the union which grouped health and social workers. [Syndicat National de la Santé et des Affaires Sociales]. It often held seminars on development issues. When we wanted to have a seminar on family planning, Ina Sissoko helped organize meetings with the women's organizations.

"To one we organized in 1970, we invited a religious leader to speak on the subject of family planning and Islam. It was a disaster. He said that even if one of his daughters would die because of an illegal abortion, he preferred that rather than family planning. Men were, in fact, the principal opponents of our efforts.

"By 1971 the idea of legalizing family planning had begun to take off despite the opposition. Sidi Coulibaly, in Social Affairs, Mme Ina and myself were all involved but Faran Samaké was the energy behind our effort.

Néné Dolo Traoré

Mme Traoré has worked as a social worker at the Malian family planning association since its creation in 1972. She interrupted her morning duties to sit with me and talk about the early days of family planning in Mali. Going beyond the past, she expressed her concern about the barriers to full reproductive freedoms which exist today.

"In the beginning the news of a family planning clinic was spread by word of mouth. All kinds of women came to us. Most of them had heard about us through the Maternal and Child Health Centres or through the maternity hospital. When they arrived we explained all the methods available, they had an examination and then chose a contraceptive method. Dr Samaké did some of the examinations but we relied mostly on midwives. Mme Ina Sissoko convinced the best known midwives of Bamako to come to the clinic. Mme Sy was in charge; she was well-known and respected by everyone. The midwives' influence was important because women knew them, many had their children delivered by them. At the outset trust was crucial to success.

"There are still many men in Mali who are opposed to their wives using a family planning method. By law women must have their husbands' permission before we can give them a contraceptive. About 95 per cent of the women in Bamako want to 'plan' but it is the husbands who sometimes object. For those who do come, either the couple comes together or the husband writes a note. If a woman comes without the husband's permission we can't help her. If we did, she would suffer at home. He wouldn't be able to do anything to us, but she might suffer the consequences. If, however, the woman is in poor health, we get a doctor's note saying that she would be in danger of grave illness if she were to become pregnant. In that case, we can help her without the husband's permission. I think women should revolt against this and see that the law is changed so that they have the right to contraceptives whether or not the husband agrees. Women must do it.

"There was a woman who came here to the clinic pregnant with her eighth child. She was extremely anaemic. We gave her a prescription and told her how important it was that she gain strength before the birth. He husband refused to pay for the medicine. She came back and she was even more anaemic and we told her what to eat and told her to sell her jewellery to buy the food she needed. She didn't dare. She died in childbirth. I learned later that her husband, to show how much he loved his wife, killed a steer for the funeral rites, to prove how much he had valued his wife... And of course, he married a new wife a few months later. Women have no value for men; he wouldn't even buy the medicine to save her.

"Men have many reasons for refusing family planning for their wives: some say it's because of religion, some say that the woman would no longer remain faithful.

"We have male clients as well, men who come to get the condom, especially young men. The condom is well accepted with the AIDS scare. There are all sorts of jokes and pet names for the condom so people are not afraid to ask for them.

"Parents bring their daughters now; that is a big change. In the beginning parents said, 'You are going to teach bad ways to our daughters'. So we didn't give contraceptives to girls less than 16 or 17 years old without a parent with her. From 17 on, she can come alone. Even that is not enough because reality is quite sad. When we made a statistical study we found that nearly 50 per cent of the girls who came to us had either had a child or an abortion already. We weren't, in fact, leading them astray; they already had lived through the consequences of their sexuality. We told their parents, 'You see, your children already know about this'.

"I don't think women's lives have improved much in the past 10 or 15 years. Women are still not free to do as they want. They have to ask men for permission to do everything, even start a small business or go to a training programme. They depend totally on the husband. In the case of divorce, men are supposed to pay for their children, but the law is not respected and how are women to go and ask the courts to help them? Even if there are laws they are not respected. Women need equality, the right to plan their families, start a business or go to school. That is what women need. A woman needs economic freedom and the right to control her own body."

Dr Faran Samaké

1932	Born Djongala, Mali
	Completed medical studies and specialization in neuro-psychiatry, University of Toulouse
	Director of the neuro-psychiatric service, Point-G Hospital, Bamako
	Invited to visit family planning programmes in Canada by CIDA
1972	Founder of the Malian Association for the Protection and Promotion of the Family (AMPPF)
1978	Died at age 46

Chapter 14
Epilogue: Looking Forward

Many lessons emerge from these recollections, and as the collector I cannot resist the opportunity to examine the messages they contain. This chapter is, thus, a very personal response to those which precede it and not all readers will agree with my views. One lesson learned from the pioneers is that they didn't always agree with each other, even though their goals were similar.

Each pioneer had a personal style of leadership. Each tackled problems in a particular way. Some chose to be out front, in the vanguard, other were "backseat" team leaders. Sensitive to the issues of ethnicity, class, medical professionalism or gender, they carefully chose the most effective approach to reach their goal.

A trait they all share is the commitment to prepare the younger generation to take over from them. Most were true mentors. They viewed planned parenthood as a broad social movement, which, to be effective, moves far beyond the medical sector. Involvement of the entire community, men, women, schools, maternal and child health services, the media and non-governmental organizations, is essential to the success of reproductive health programmes.

Voluntary organizations were a formidable force in shaping government policies. Volunteer groups pushed governments to undertake family planning programmes and set high standards for government services. In the case of Bangladesh, Tunisia and Ghana, government family planning programmes benefitted directly from volunteer efforts by subsequently hiring founder members of family planning associations to direct government initiatives.

Conferences and study tours were very effective tools in spreading the word about planned parenthood, contraceptive technologies and in encouraging individuals who needed intellectual and moral support for their work. Also, the visits of Margaret Sanger, Senator Kato and staff members of The Pathfinder Fund, the Population Council, or other such groups

172

were catalysts for local action. Those who were unable to travel abroad or have access to the latest information and technologies benefited greatly from these contacts, as did the visitors themselves.

It appears that the women pioneers reached out to a wide support group to pursue their goals. The men, all medical doctors, were more narrowly focused. It may be that when women are involved in the design and implementation of programmes, those programmes are broader and more sensitive to women's needs.

Nearly every individual interviewed for this volume voiced concern about the lack of sex education. They told of the difficulties of promoting sexual health and planned parenthood when few people had any notion of their anatomy or reproductive cycles. Several women stated that they had never been told about menstruation and were totally surprised, some frightened, when they first discovered their menstrual blood. Elsie Locke noted, with frustration, "Family planning came to be accepted long before sex education." The taboo surrounding sexuality had, and continues to have, frightening consequences.

But beyond the work documented here lie insights into the biases of the medical profession, into how negligent we have been in educating the young for full and healthy sexuality, and into the way society views and treats its women. This last observation is, in my view, the most significant for guiding future efforts.Certainly it is clear from the proceeding chapters that family planning is an essential component of maternal and child health. Without access to safe contraceptives and quality counselling, women and girls easily fall victim to unplanned pregnancies, anaemia and fatigue, infection and unsafe abortions. Certainly it is clear also, that without access to the means to voluntary motherhood, women will live in constant fear of unwanted pregnancy. As a young wife, living in a country where contraceptives were illegal, I suffered that fear. It is all consuming. Every month I hoped, even prayed, that I would escape a pregnancy I did not want and which my husband, who took no precautions, did not want. Too young and ill-informed to make demands, I simply endured the fear. Thirty-five years later there are hundreds of millions of women who experience that same fear each month. What is often left unsaid is that abortions to please a husband are very common. And in cases where a husband forbids a wife's use of contraceptives, regardless of her health or wishes, unsafe abortion may be her only recourse.

In Senator Shidzue Kato's words, if women are not allowed the knowledge (and means) to control their bodies, they will never be free. This freedom to which she alludes may be why there is such opposition to reproductive freedom. Why else would we be witnessing attempts to curtail the basic human right of women to planned motherhood in this last decade of the 20th century? I truly believe that opposition to planned parenthood takes its origin in profound misogyny and fear of women. If women are able to decide if and when they will become mothers, they are far more self-confident. With self-confidence comes independent decision-making and participation in the life of society. As a disinherited group, women's claim to economic and political power threatens those who now hold it.

Women only learned how disinherited they are through the vast data gathering effort undertaken at the time of International Women's Year and the UN Decade for Women (1975–85) which followed. Until then, little was known of the lives of the unseen, unheard women of the world. Suddenly the double standard in rights, health, access to education, training and equal pay was clearly documented. Domestic violence, forced marriages, harmful traditional practices were exposed for the world to see. And women saw and heard each other. Concern for the abysmal status of women resulted in the *UN Convention on the Elimination of All Forms of Discrimination Against Women*. One hundred and seven nations have signed the convention since its adoption in 1979. But the backlash has been significant. When women began to demand their rights, they were blamed for an increase in divorce rates and contraceptives were seen as part of "the problem". There was a concerted campaign to trivialize women's demands and to discredit women's rights activists, feminists, pro-choice groups and women leaders.

The reality of women's lives reveals that in many societies girl children are denied, from infancy onward, full personhood by custom, status and lack of access to education and medical care. Married at an early age, they pass from one man's domination to another man's control. One might suppose, then, that women are well cared for. Not so. One third of all households in the world are headed by women due to migration, divorce or abandonment. Research shows that households headed by women are the poorest, their children the least advantaged. Violence against women is endemic in all societies. Hidden, barely discussed, but frequent, it is a cancer eating away at the will and dignity of women and at their ability to make decisions for themselves. In Peru, 70 per cent of all crimes reported to the police involve women being beaten by their partners![1] Parental preference for male children is widespread. It is estimated that neglect of and discrimination against female children leads to serious health consequences which account for between 500,000 and 1 million deaths per annum among female children.[2]

According to the Population Reference Bureau a total of 33 per cent of the world's population is currently under the age of 15. The large cities of the world are host to a nomadic population of "street children" numbering in the tens of millions from Calcutta to New York, from Sao Paulo to Nairobi. Boys and girls, forced to live by their wits, sleeping in squalor and insecurity, have little access to services or assistance. They have little choice but to turn to crime and prostitution to survive. Cast aside by society, they are the parents of tomorrow – and today. Adolescents give birth to one in every seven babies born in the Western Hemisphere. Between 80 and 90 births per thousand are born to adolescents in Latin America, compared to 51 in Canada.[3]   Nafis Sadik, the leader of the UN Population Fund, gives us good advice: "The challenge for those who believe that women's contribution is central to development – and that investment in women should take priority, even in societies under severe economic stress – is to make an *irresistible case for change*."[4] To make that case the true status of women, of women's health *and the barriers they confront* must be central to planning and programme design and that will necessitate that governments rethink the value they give their womenfolk. Too often women's needs are dismissed as peripheral, and appear last on the list of funding priorities.

The women who are profiled in this book are examples of what happens when girls and women are supported by families and society, allowed to study and participate in the public domain. Their experience also demonstrates that women listen to women, are close to women's needs: a clear call for women's leadership in the social issues of our time.

The experts say that women's education is a crucial factor in decreasing family size. That may be true statistically, but it is also true that in most families it is men who approve the use of a contraceptive. Common sense has little to do with literacy; when a woman – educated or not – knows the family's resources are stretched to the limit, she knows she does not need another child to feed. But, they say, "My husband doesn't understand".[5] Educating men and boys about responsible fatherhood seems not only logical but a question of fundamental justice. By the same token, we might educate our male politicians about responsible leadership, which recognizes women's contributions to society and their claim to full partnership in that society.

A recent survey of the voting records of members of the House and Senate in the US Congress shows that "members of Congress who vote to keep abortion legal and available are the same members, by and large, who vote to create conditions that welcome childbearing and child-rearing. Conversely, those members who oppose legal abortion also tend to vote against a range of policies supporting human life, including those which assist women in securing the resources and services they need once they choose to have children".[6] Given facts such as these, one must ask: Is this debate about abortion or about controlling women? The pioneers quoted here were vilified for proposing voluntary motherhood, planned families. They held fast. The right to planned parenthood is now enshrined in international law. Abortion is the last stand, the smoke-screen behind which conservative forces hide in their attempt to prevent women's full participation in society.

The pioneer advocates of planned parenthood were, years ago, horrified by the results of failed contraception or the lack of contraceptive services. Today, non-medical abortion remains one of the greatest plagues of our society. Hundreds of thousands of women and girls die each year as a result of their society's refusal to provide early safe, abortion. It is estimated that one woman dies in childbirth, or due to pregnancy-related causes each minute. Half of them die of non-medical abortions. Failure to address this health crisis is irresponsible, if not worse. "In Latin American and the Caribbean, childbearing and abortion are among the five principal causes of death for 15 to 19 year old females. In Argentina, Chile, Colombia, Guyana and Trinidad and Tobago, unsafe abortion is responsible for one quarter of maternal deaths and in Paraguay it is responsible for two-thirds of those deaths."[7] Prohibition of abortion does not prevent it, but kills women. Good reproductive care requires *a combination* of safe contraceptives and medically-supervised abortion. Legalized abortion without access to contraceptives, such as Miyoshi Ohba encountered in post-war Japan, is foolish. In the case of failed contraception, early abortion is essential to comprehensive family planning. Indeed, as Jodi Jacobson demonstrates so clearly, "Without access to abortion, it is impossible for a woman to have total control over her own fertility".[8]

Miyoshi Ohba pointed out that it takes two partners to produce a child or to avoid a pregnancy; her recognition of that simple fact led her to create the Mandarin Duck Club over 40 years ago. Reliable contraception and the partner's co-operation are the only means of avoiding an unwanted pregnancy. If either fail, the woman pays the price. She has two choices: either she gives birth to and cares for the unwanted child, or she takes the risk of terminating the pregnancy. The male partner, the religious or legal authorities, have no responsibility to feed, love, care for, support that undesired child. Who, then, should make the decision? And if the woman chooses to assure that all her children are wanted children, should she not have proper abortion facilities available to her? The respect of individual rights to privacy and self determination is one of the corner stones of democratic societies. The tradition of secular states has been to separate religious beliefs from the law. That tradition is currently undergoing a challenge from conservative religious groups which seek to impose their views. The anti-choice movement is exporting its propaganda worldwide.

The International Youth Pro-Life Federation has trained foreign students to build anti-choice movements in their nations when they return home. They describe family planners as "racists", "murderers, "anti-family", "promoters of promiscuity" – and even proposed that they are "anti-children", a supposition which made New Zealander Elsie Locke laugh aloud 40 years ago.

Faced with the controversy surrounding family planning and abortion, government leadership has often failed to uphold reproductive rights and services. Over the past 5–10 years we have seen political leaders become evasive, dodging the issue or, worse still, changing their votes to please the opposition to women's reproductive freedom. But in denying access to modern contraception or to abortion is a denial of human rights law. Indeed, it is an abrogation of the basic human right to have the information and the means to "decide freely and responsibly on the number and spacing of their children".

With the remarkable breakthrough drug, RU 486, abortion becomes far less invasive, more private and less dangerous. Yet again we have witnessed conservative groups damning its sale and use. When the Roussel-Uclaf drug company bowed to their pressure and announced it would suspend marketing of the drug, the French Health Minister, Claude Evin, ordered it back on the market stating that RU 486 is "the moral property of women, not just the property of the drug company". This precedent of official enlightenment is a sign that there still are risk takers, new pioneers of reproductive freedoms. It also demonstrates, alas, that women's well-being is dependent upon that enlightenment.

Today's pioneers, like those before them, are willing to take risks, defy bureaucracies and laws to guarantee rights, broaden services and increase opportunities for women and their families. They have created women's health co-operatives, rape crisis centres and homes for battered women. They campaign against the multi-billion dollar sex-ploitation business and assist young women who manage to escape its grasp. They work to eradicate female genital mutilation and traditions like Devadasi dedication[9]. Others denounce double standards in education, health and legal status which women have endured for centuries. The new pioneers are breaking away from the medical monopoly on pregnancy and motherhood, helping women to retrieve their birthing process from doctor-centered care. They promote home birthing, the legal recognition of midwifery, the expansion of natural childbirth.

In a world where between 9 and 11 million are believed to be infected with HIV (WHO) and in which there are 10,000 new AIDS sufferers per month, new pioneers work in a range of AIDS prevention initiatives. They are working to expand health care training and services available to women. They believe that family planning and HIV prevention education should go hand in hand. Their work includes assisting prostitutes and street children. When Evangelina Rodriguez began her work with prostitutes, she was condemned for social misbehaviour. Today it is prostitutes who are educating their clients about HIV.

One cannot help but see the similarities between the experiences of early family planners and those spearheading AIDS prevention work. The subject of AIDS unsettles people just as the question of birth control did years ago for it touches upon human sexual relations. Political leaders tend to deny its danger, to dismiss it as something which does not affect all populations. As with any crisis which is denied at the outset, over-reaction later is the danger. Loss of civil liberties and discriminatory practices may well be the norm if the

AIDS pandemic is left to spread by passive denial. Leaving the fight against AIDS to the medical community would be foolish: just as in family planning, the involvement of the entire community, including schools and non-governmental institutions is an essential element in transmitting knowledge and changing behaviour.

Thailand's creative and well-known family planner, Mechai Viravaidya, has understood this connection and is currently designing an AIDS prevention effort focused on the sex trade. Tourism has become Thailand's major source of foreign exchange, earning nearly $4 billion in 1989.[10] But beyond this, studies reveal that four to six million Thai men visit a prostitute at least once a month.[11] In a country where an estimated 300,000 Thais are HIV positive, Thai women, married or unmarried, must learn to protect themselves to prevent HIV contamination. We can no longer separate family planning from sexuality, sexual health and sex education; we can no longer separate prevention of sexually transmitted diseases from family planning. With the HIV pandemic, we will have to be honest and compassionate about human sexuality if we are to protect each other from certain death.

New pioneers are involved in advocacy work, broadening legislation, monitoring changes in family law, contraceptive safety and lobbying government for enlightened reproductive health policies. The recent case of Planned Parenthood Federation of America *versus* the Government of the United States is another example of more active advocacy of reproductive freedoms. Recently, Dr Fred Sai, President of the International Planned Parenthood Federation, sought a dialogue with the Vatican. In a letter addressed to the Pope dated 11 July 1991, Dr Sai wrote, "I humbly suggest that a sensitive dialogue should be opened between the Church and those who believe as I do that voluntary family planning is the best protection against abortion, as well as a major contributor to saving women's lives and a human right." *The National Catholic Register* carried a story on Dr Sai's letter saying, "But a Vatican spokesman said bluntly that John Paul II will not respond to the letter, and that the whole matter was not something to be taken seriously by the Holy See."[12] The Pope resists attempts within the Church itself to relax restrictions on contraceptive use.

New pioneers are following the footsteps of Ottar Ottesen-Jensen to expand sex education, knowledge related to sexuality, reproductive health and family planning. In many societies incest, child abuse, wife rape and violence against women are far more readily discussed than healthy, non-exploitative sexuality. Sexual "literacy" which eradicates taboos, misinformation and encourages sexual health is and will continue to be, a controversial subject. Yet its benefits are obvious: in countries like Holland which has the lowest incidence of teenage pregnancy and abortion in the world, sex education begins in early childhood. The tragic reality of adolescent pregnancies might be avoided if sex education began at an early age, if quality counselling and contraceptive services for adolescents were more readily available.

As before, pioneering initiatives come from individuals or from groups. Volunteer, non-governmental organizations are becoming a powerful force for influencing public policy. Yet there is a danger that success may turn them into just another bureaucracy. Julia Henderson, former Secretary General of IPPF, commented on the current volunteer situation in family planning associations, "In many countries the volunteers seem to have been there forever. This is why I feel that it's really time for a change of generations."[13] Singapore's Constance Goh agrees and calls for a renewal of the volunteer spirit, "The family planning movement is top heavy now, a lot of bureaucracy and waste. There is room for a lot of improvement, more zeal, more commitment. My experience shows that women started the family planning movement at the ground level and then, when it became respectable, the men jumped in. We need more women at all levels and especially up the hierarchy."

As I travelled to collect the interviews of pioneers, I rarely found women in positions of decision-making in the family planning associations. In fact, in one country, when I attempted to question a woman fieldworker about her work, the male supervisor insisted on answering the questions. This incident reminds me of the past 20 years of development programmes where predominantly male planners, managers and experts considered the illiterate "target populations" of development projects to be so lacking in common sense that they didn't bother to consult them about their needs.

Taboos, customs and laws still have to be eradicated or changed before all women will have the right to choose if and when to be a mother. In my view the first step in that effort entails exposing the shameful double standards with which the world community, and its governments, treat its women.

The management of women's reproductive and productive

lives takes place in obscure, insidious ways. There where the state wants more workers or soldiers, it adopts a pro-natalist policy. When population expansion is too fast, suddenly disincentives to women's labour and education appear. Everywhere women's labour is exploited: as unpaid agricultural and domestic workers or as underpaid contributors to national economies. Powerful financial interests abuse women's bodies as "executive entertainment" and tourist bait. Indeed, the double standard is a profitable convenience. While extolling the virtues of Motherhood and "woman's destiny", leaders of nations, religions and institutions look the other way while millions of women's lives are dominated by violence, abandonment, lack of education, training, lack of child support and child care.

The new pioneers tell us there is a long way to go in the effort to assure full and healthy lives for women and girls, to guarantee the right to choose safe and healthy motherhood. The experience of the older pioneers demonstrates we can't wait for someone else to do it for us.

References

1. *Women in the World*, an International Atlas, Page 102.
2. UNECOSOC Commission on Human Rights E/CN.4/1986/42.
3. Singh, Susheela and Deidre Wulf, *Today's Adolescents: Tomorrow's parents: A Portrait of the Americas* (The Alan Guttmacher Institute, 1991).
4. Nafis Sadik, *Investing in Women: the Focus of the Nineties* UNFPA, *State of World Population*, 1989.
5. Huston, Perdita, *Message From the Village* (New York: UNFPA and the Epoch B Foundation, 1979).
6. *Actions Speak Louder*, A look at Congressional Votes on Human Life Issues, CONSCIENCE, Catholics for a Free Choice, Washington, DC, 1991.
7. *Adolescent Pregnancy in Latin America and the Caribbean*, a brochure, IPPF Western Hemisphere Region, 1988.
8. Jacobson, Jodi L., Worldwatch Paper 97, *The Global Politics of Abortion*, July 1990, Washington DC page 49.
9. ISIS-WICCE, *Women's World*, No 24, winter 1990-1991 page 28. Dedicated to the Goddess Yellamma at the time of puberty, sold in auction, these young girls can no longer be married and by religion are obliged to amuse men in order to receive Yellamma's benediction. These girls account for an average 15 per cent of the prostitutes of India and up to 80 per cent of those living in the southern regions of the country.
10. *Thailand, Burma Country Profile, 1990-1991*, Annual survey of Political and Economic Background, The Economist Intelligence Unit, London, 1990.
11. *Thai Development Newsletter*, November 19, 1990, Thai Development Support Committee.
12. National Catholic Register, *IPPF Overture meets with Dead Silence*, 11 August, 1991.
13. *Revitalizing FPA*, JOICFP NEWS, August 1991.

BIBLIOGRAPHY

Britannica, *Micropaedia Ready Reference* (1985).

Dobbie, Marie, *A Matter for Women*, The New Zealand Family Planning Association 1936 to 1976, as yet unpublished.

Goh Kok Kee, Constance, *Reminiscence of Early Family Planning Days in Singapore and South East Asia*, Study Group Presentation, 21-24 September 1983.

International Planned Parenthood Federation, *Planned Parenthood in Europe*, Vol 18, No 1.

JOICFP, *Where There is a Will, The Story of a Countryside Health Nurse* JOICFP Document Series 3 (Tokyo 1981).

Kato, Shidzue, *A Fight for Women's Happiness, Pioneering the Family Planning Movement in Japan*, JOICFP Document Series 11 (Tokyo, 1984).

Law, M., Maine, D. and Feuerstein, M-T, *Safe Motherhood: Priorities and Next Steps*, UN Development Programme, April 1991.

Locke, Elsie, *Birth Control: A Women's Achievement*, Race, Gender, Class. No 3, July 1986.

Locke, Elsie, *Student at the Gates*, (Christchurch: Whitcoulls Publishers, 1981).

Ministry of Information, *Facts About Bangladesh*, Government of the People's Republic of Bangladesh, (1989).

Patterson, Kim, *I can't go on having child after child. . .*", *New Zealand Women's Weekly*, October 6, 1986.

Stiernborg, Leila, *Ottar Fund*, PEOPLE, Vol 13, No 2 1986.

Suitters, Beryl, *Be Brave and Angry*, Chronicles of the International Planned Parenthood Federation (London: IPPF, 1973).

Zaglul, Antonio, *Despreciada en la Vida y Olvidada en la Muerte* Biografia de Evangelina Rodriguez, la Primera medica Dominicana (Santo Domingo: Editora Taller, DR 1980).